CODE OF PRACTICE FOR DISABILITY EQUIPMENT, WHEELCHAIR AND SEATING SERVICES

A QUALITY FRAMEWORK FOR PROCUREMENT AND PROVISION OF SERVICES

UNITED KINGDOM

CODE OF PRACTICE FOR DISABILITY EQUIPMENT, WHEELCHAIR AND SEATING SERVICES

A QUALITY FRAMEWORK FOR PROCUREMENT AND PROVISION OF SERVICES

UNITED KINGDOM

BRIAN DONNELLY

Published by:
Community Equipment Solutions Ltd
71 Church Street
Great Missenden
Buckinghamshire HP16 0AZ
E: info@communityequipment.org.uk
W: www.communityequipment.org.uk

in association with
Matador
9 Priory Business Park
Wistow Road
Kibworth
Leics LE8 0RX
www.troubador.co.uk

British Library Cataloguing in Publication Data. A catalogue record for this book is available from the British Library.

Printed and bound in the UK by TJ International Ltd, Padstow, Cornwall.

ISBN 9781784623029

Matador is an imprint of Troubador Publishing Ltd

CODE OF PRACTICE FOR DISABILITY EQUIPMENT, WHEELCHAIR AND SEATING SERVICES

A QUALITY FRAMEWORK FOR PROCUREMENT AND PROVISION OF SERVICES

UNITED KINGDOM

Contents

Forewords

Baroness Grey-Thompson DBE, DL

I am delighted to have been asked to give a foreword to this Code of Practice for disability equipment, wheelchair and seating services, for many reasons. In fact, I am very encouraged that it has been written at all.

From a young age I have used a range of disability equipment and wheelchairs, so I know first-hand what it is like to be on the receiving end of services, both good and bad. Some people may have read about my frustrations in my 'tweets' when I have to crawl up and down stairs when my lift is broken, or when there is no access on and off trains!

I had an independent streak even at a very young age, and having equipment was essential to enable me to achieve my ambitions.

Disability equipment is often associated with the medical model of care. Obviously this is important, but just focussing on a medical condition can blinker the overall assessment, and not allow for wider aspirations and lifestyle choices. Of course there are different organisations and services involved in providing equipment, and I am glad to see this Code addresses this key issue by promoting integration and the social model of disability.

Equipment can allow people to access the curriculum, work, sport and leisure. Getting the right equipment in itself can remove many barriers to independence and inclusion.

Equipment has evolved incredibly since I started using it and without it I may not have achieved my lifelong ambitions in sport. In the twenty-first century, there is a vast range of technology available to enhance the life experiences of disabled people; we need to deploy it more smartly so that we can unleash the potential and ambitions of many people.

An important factor for me when growing up and being assessed was being listened to. I usually got the equipment I needed in the end, but it was not always without a fight. Disabled people should not have to fight for basic aids to give them the same opportunities as others. I am encouraged to see this Code actively promotes and encourages service users and their carers to be involved at every level.

I like the idea of having outcome-based standards, as set out in this Code, mainly because it starts to provide a standard we can all work to and can expect, without being too prescriptive about how everything should be done. I also like the fact that it has a UK-wide focus.

The forty-seven 'bite-size' Code Standards break down what is otherwise a very complex system into something manageable and understandable. It is also encouraging to see that the Code draws on relevant legislation like, for example, the UN Convention on the Rights of Disabled People, making sure hard fought for and won legislative change filters through to ground level.

However optimistic and committed governments and organisations are to improving outcomes for disabled people, practical steps are required to make these improvements; I believe this Code lays down steps that need to be taken. Let's just hope it is followed!

Baroness Grey-Thompson DBE, DL
Baroness Grey-Thompson, DBE, DL, is a British former wheelchair racer and is a parliamentarian. She is considered to be one of the most successful disabled athletes in the UK. Over her career she won a total of sixteen Paralympic medals, including eleven golds, held over thirty world records and won the London Marathon six times between 1992 and 2002. In 1993 she was appointed Member of the Order of the British Empire (MBE) for 'services to sport', advanced in 2000 to OBE again for 'services to sport' and then in 2005 was promoted to Dame Commander of the Order of the British Empire (DBE). In 2010 Tanni was appointed to the House of Lords, where she serves as a non-party political crossbench peer. Tanni took the title Baroness Grey-Thompson of Eaglescliffe in the County of Durham.

Sir Bert Massie CBE, DL

As someone who has been disabled for almost all of my life and a user of a wide range of disability equipment, I am delighted to welcome this new Code of Practice for disability equipment, wheelchair and seating services.

I have been involved in disability issues for over forty-five years and believe the development of the new Code takes significant steps towards improving people's experience of private and statutory provision of wheelchairs and disability equipment. The Code sets a national (UK), and perhaps international, benchmark against which services can be measured, and sets a realistic level of service people should expect to receive – something that has been missing for a long time.

A disabled person often uses a range of disability equipment, e.g. wheelchair, speech-board, telecare, hoist, handrails, ramps and many other items. Yet these items are often provided by different departments or statutory bodies, which can cause delays and stress for service users, as well as unnecessary cost, time and effort to the staff and organisations providing the equipment. Integration is essential to improve user experience and simultaneously create efficiencies by streamlining services. This Code breaks new ground as it not only promotes integration of services, but also shows how to do it. It also pioneers the concept of holistic assessments, which are essential for the delivery of true person-centred care. The Code supports all models of provision, and provides the necessary safeguards for each.

Working with the new Code paves the way for reducing the administration of services, with the associated delays and waste – aims governments everywhere should embrace wholeheartedly. There needs to be an overall strategy for the full range of disability equipment and assistive technologies, and the Code is a ready-made template to support this.

To make any lasting and meaningful improvements, we need to understand and to be able to measure the demand for services, ensure funding matches that demand, and that equipment-related services are appropriately commissioned in an integrated way that allows for a holistic and person-centred approach. This needs to be supported by having clear and realistic specifications in place, and competent staff to deliver the service. Crucially, users and their carers need to be involved all along the way.

We must also be able to measure and report on the success of having a good service, i.e. outcomes, not just statistics, and ensure any success factors are sustainable and able to withstand changes in government policy or demographics. Following this new Code of Practice will help in achieving these aims.

The Code of Practice rightly starts with the service user, and looks into services from the outside. It strongly recommends the involvement of service users and their carers. Disabled people are not fools and nor should we be passive recipients of services provided by professionals. The force of user involvement is something that has not yet been fully harnessed and utilised in the development of these services. This is where real changes can be made. I therefore welcome the parts of the Code that refer to and strongly recommend user involvement.

For many of us disability is not an event but a long-term feature of our lives. We know that a short-term solution can often have long-term consequences that cost more to manage than could ever be saved by the cost conscious short-term solution. Getting services right in the future begins now. The work of the Code looks long-term and that must be right.

Quite simply, the Code of Practice is an essential tool to support central and local governments, commissioners, providers and clinical teams alike, and working with the Code will ensure the service user gets the outcomes we all want to see.

As this new Code spans across a range of disability equipment and assistive technology-related services, including wheelchair and seating, and across all sectors, it will play an important role in supporting seamless care pathways, paving the way for true integration and breaking down the artificial and long-standing silos between services and organisations – something that needs to happen if we really want to address the funding crisis and support disabled and elderly people.

I cannot think of one reason why organisations and people everywhere wouldn't want to follow this Code. Can you?

Sir Bert Massie CBE, DL
Sir Bert Massie CBE, DL, is the Chairman of CECOPS CIC, a UK-based standards body for disability equipment services. Sir Bert has had senior roles in the past including being Chairman of the Disability Rights Commission, and Chief Executive of the Royal Association for Disability and Rehabilitation (RADAR). He was appointed a CBE in 2000 and knighted in 2007.

Preface

This new edition follows on naturally from the previous *Code of Practice for Community Equipment (2011)*; it is the logical next step. Again it sets out forty-seven outcome-based Code Standards, covering the commissioning, provision and clinical aspects of services. This edition has a UK-wide focus and as well as covering disability equipment services, it now incorporates wheelchair and seating services; it also provides strong links to all other assistive technology-related services so that person-centred and holistic care can be provided. The outcome-based standards included within this Code are written in such a way that they can also be applied internationally.

Although daunted by the prospect of having to write another Code of Practice, I felt I had no option as I was constantly asked by people all across the UK (and other parts of the world), when I was planning to write a Code to include wheelchair and seating services. Clearly there was a need for standards in these key services, and there was certainly a demand from the ground, so I had no option but to put pen to paper.

The Code of Practice can be used by anyone or any organisation involved in the commissioning or provision of disability equipment, or in making clinical assessments for this equipment; it is also the official reference guide for CECOPS' registration and accreditation scheme, which you are welcome to join. Visit www.cecops.org.uk for more information.

One of the key aims of this updated Code is to promote person-centred care, a term we often hear about, and nowhere is it more necessary than in the provision of disability equipment and assistive technology services. I have used the term 'holistic assessments' because I feel that it is at the root of improving user experience, and is crucial to the achievement of better outcomes and true person-centred care: treating each service user as one person with a range of needs, which statutory bodies must aim to meet as seamlessly as possible.

Service users often need to access the full range of equipment services, but these usually have different commissioning and assessment arrangements. This makes it difficult for them to navigate their way through the system, and also means that they have a number of different contacts and assessments. The result is duplication, delay and dissatisfied service users. This needs to change at organisational level: in particular, commissioners need to recognise how much they could achieve by embracing integration and forging links with other organisations and departments working in the same sphere. Whilst changes won't happen overnight, this Code of Practice sets the ball rolling by giving commissioners a template to work to when procuring these services, and making sure they understand and think about what they are asking providers to do.

Following this Code will help to provide seamless and good quality care for service users when they need it. It will help everyone to understand more clearly the different aspects of commissioning and provision, and what standard of service should be provided. Following the Code also enables organisations and staff to meet all their relevant legal and regulatory obligations in one place.

I don't really like talking about money in the same breath as talking about improving the quality of services and outcomes, but I firmly believe, and there are many pieces of evidence to support this view, that providing the right equipment in a timely way results in significant savings, mainly through the avoidance of secondary and unnecessary episodes of care, e.g. hospital admissions. Following this Code will greatly help in realising these benefits – a win-win really!

Enabling more people to be independent, and have more choice and control over their own care, are stated government priorities, and there is great scope for this where disability equipment is concerned. But there need to be mechanisms and safeguards in place to ensure this happens safely and effectively, and this Code provides practical steps towards achievement of these priorities.

I am often asked why I am so interested in this particular area of care, and why I wanted to develop standards. I have worked in these services for a long time, and seeing the difference a piece of equipment can make to someone's life is truly inspiring. To see the smile on a child's face because he or she can walk or get around, or seeing someone able to communicate, where before they couldn't, is a delight to witness. I can remember a mother saying to me that for years she pushed her daughter in a manual wheelchair and was never able to walk down the street holding her hand like other mothers; but she was able to after her daughter received a powered wheelchair. It might sound like a small thing, but these things matter to individuals in their daily lives; getting lots of small things right, together makes a big difference, and these small achievements wouldn't happen without having the right services in place.

I have also been motivated by witnessing cases where people with rapidly progressing conditions or terminal illnesses can't get the equipment they need to support them in their remaining days, to die at home or to be able to communicate. These are some of the examples that have motivated me to write standards for these essential services. One day I might need the services myself, and I would want to be assured that I got the right equipment in a timely way, from someone competent to carry out my assessment. I am amazed no one has undertaken this work before, given the enormity of the need and the benefits these services can bring.

I am under no illusion that by following this Code all the difficulties associated with commissioning and providing disability equipment and wheelchair and seating services will be addressed, but I am certain it will significantly improve overall outcomes for organisations and service users.

Lastly, I sincerely hope the Code and the principles set out within it are followed, not only in the UK but all across the world.

Brian Donnelly MSc

Acknowledgements

The author would like to thank the following individuals and organisations:

My wife, Naomi, for fully supporting me in everything I do. Sir Bert Massie CBE, DL, for his long-standing and continued support. Baroness Tanni Grey-Thompson DBE, DL, for her support and for taking the time to provide a foreword for this Code. Krys Jarvis, Chair of National Wheelchair Managers' Forum (NWMF), and other members of NWMF who contributed supporting information. Gail Russell, WPMS Ltd and Sarah Clayton, Postural Care CIC, for their ongoing support and encouragement. Karen Pearce, Motor Neurone Disease Association, for her public support for this work. Liam Dwyer, a friend and a sufferer of Motor Neurone Disease, for his enthusiastic and public support for this work, and for giving permission to use his image on the front cover of the Code. Dr Sue Hurrell and her daughter Imogen for giving permission to use a lovely picture of Imogen on the cover of the Code. Lastly, to all the other individuals and organisations that have provided 'moral' support to write this new Code.

Overview of the Code of Practice

This new edition of the Code of Practice applies to all disability equipment, wheelchair and seating services in the UK and, except for the UK legislation in Appendix 1, in other parts of the world. It supersedes the original and successful *Code of Practice for Community Equipment (2011)*. Again it is a quality framework for the procurement and provision of services.

The Code of Practice sets the benchmark and standard that services everywhere should be aspiring to.

For those planning, designing or commissioning services, this Code of Practice provides a template for ensuring all risks, governance, quality and health and safety duties, obligations and standards are clearly specified within service specifications issued to providers. It is also a useful tool for managing provider performance.

For providers and clinical staff, the Code sets out the standard of service which should be provided, and acts as a guide for monitoring and assessing overall performance of the service provided. It also allows the provider to demonstrate the quality and performance of their services.

The Code of Practice and CECOPS CIC

The Code of Practice is the official reference guide for CECOPS' registration and accreditation scheme. CECOPS CIC is a UK-based independent not-for-profit standards body; it is supported by regulators, professional bodies and a range of other organisations.

Details about how the scheme works, including registration and accreditation, can be found on the CECOPS website here:

www.cecops.org.uk, or for more information contact here: info@cecops.org.uk

The Code of Practice can be used either as part of CECOPS or as a standalone reference guide.

The Code of Practice aligns with current legislative and regulatory obligations in the UK.

How to use the Code of Practice and CECOPS

Commissioners are expected to work to the specific standards in Parts 1 and 4 of the Code, relating to their activities. In addition, they can include compliance with the Code as a requirement within appropriate procurement/tendering documentation. The most common use in this respect is for commissioners to require providers, including clinical teams, to be registered with CECOPS and to become accredited post contract award. Accreditation involves an external assessment which is undertaken by highly qualified quality and risk management assessors.

Providers work to Part 2 of the Code, supplemented by any Code Standards within Part 4 that are relevant to their activities. Clinical teams, or independent clinical practitioners, work to Part 3 of the Code, again supplemented where necessary by Code Standards selected from Part 4.

Whether requested by the commissioner or not, providers, including clinical teams, can register with CECOPS and seek to become accredited. Many providers choose to do this to demonstrate their good quality service and high standards, or as a tool to help drive continuous improvement. It is also used to help manage services, proactively. Some providers work with the Code and CECOPS to seek competitive advantage over competitors.

Organisations with both commissioning and provider responsibilities can work to all Parts of the Code of Practice.

Benefits of working with the Code of Practice

Where the Code is closely followed, it provides the following benefits:

- getting the right equipment at the right time, with improved outcomes;
- helps to achieve strategic and policy objectives;
- involves service users in decisions and service design, which raises satisfaction levels;
- enables safer and better quality services by providing a framework to work to, and a national benchmark for assessing standard and performance levels of services;
- enables legal, regulatory, welfare duties and obligations to be met in one place;
- provides a ready-made template for commissioners and providers;
- supports seamless care pathways across equipment-related services;
- generates efficiencies by avoiding costlier secondary episodes of care, and smarter procurement;
- provides a tool for managing contracts;
- provides assurance that staff at all levels are competent;
- allows quality improvements to be driven at local level;
- supports all service delivery models and provides safeguards;
- provides quality of life for the service user by also regarding social model of disability and 'whole-life' needs;
- addresses historic concerns and recommendations from previous disability equipment and wheelchair service reviews;
- helps achieve a variety of care-related policies and strategies, e.g. early intervention, prevention, enablement;
- improves early years development for disabled children;
- reduces risk and likelihood of unnecessary injuries, e.g. falls, pressure ulcers, untoward incidents and fatalities;
- cuts unscheduled hospital admissions, and avoids crisis admissions to high-cost services;
- reduces length of hospital stay and 'bed blocking';
- enables timely discharge from hospital and supports post-discharge recovery;
- provides seamless care pathway for service users across different care agencies;

- supports carers and parents in managing care needs and well-being;
- keeps more people independent in the community, and
- assists with funding of long-term care.

Important points to note

Understanding the Parts of the Code
The Code of Practice contains forty-seven Code Standards; not all of these will be relevant to each organisation. The Code consists of three main Parts covering commissioning, service provision and clinical responsibilities respectively, together with a fourth supplementary Part. Organisations can use some or all of the Parts, depending on what is relevant to their activities. For example, a disability equipment store may only need to use Part 2, but some wheelchair and seating services with both a store and in-house clinical staff may need to use Parts 2 and 3. In addition to the main applicable Part, any relevant Code Standards in the supplementary Part 4 should also be worked to. It is left to the judgement and discretion of the organisation which of the standards in any Part to apply to their service.

Understanding outcomes and clauses
You will notice that each Code Standard has an outcome; this is the wording set out in the shaded box. This is ultimately the outcome you are expected to work to and against which you would be assessed if you chose to become accredited. Below the outcome is a series of clauses. The clauses set out ways in which you could achieve the outcome. However, you may have alternative measures in place to meet the outcome, and this is perfectly acceptable. The clauses are not absolute requirements.

Understanding terminology
Throughout this Code of Practice the term 'equipment' relates to disability equipment and wheelchair and seating products. The terms 'equipment service' or just 'service' relate to disability equipment services and wheelchair and seating services, unless otherwise stated.

The use of the title 'Service User'
There are numerous titles given to describe people that use the various

equipment services, e.g. service user, citizen, client and patient. Different individuals and organisations have their own preferred titles. Whilst we respect this and have no preferred title, for consistency we have used the term 'service user' throughout this Code and we sincerely hope this doesn't offend any particular client group or individual.

Introduction

The growing elderly population is a global trend which, coupled with an increase in the number of people living with Long-Term Conditions (LTCs), increases demand for health and care services, with associated fiscal strains, in all societies.

Continuing with the same models of delivery is not going to be sustainable. New approaches and service delivery models need to be found that will deliver more efficient and effective care, whilst maintaining safe and good quality services.

People need to be equipped with the right products and services to help them become more independent and to be better supported in managing their own care. This includes disabled children and adults, to ensure they have the same life expectations, opportunities and outcomes as other citizens. Services also need to be geared toward prevention and early intervention to avoid unnecessary and costlier episodes of care later on.

One method to address some of the concerns above is the better deployment of assistive technologies – from walking aids, beds, wheelchairs, and communication aids, through to more advanced electronic assistive technologies such as telecare products and telehealth equipment. If used strategically these can support health and care services significantly and meet a range of government policy aims.

Not only does effective provision of assistive technology improve outcomes for service users, including social inclusion and quality of life, but it can also reduce the burden on the state by enabling independent living, enhancing employment prospects and enabling individuals to take control of their own lives – all of which have a part to play in tackling the worldwide problem of funding longevity.

But a shift towards better deployment of all assistive technologies has not really happened at scale, for a variety of reasons. At strategic level, there is generally failure to appreciate the benefits of this equipment, and as a result there is no overall strategy or vision to integrate the many departments and bodies which currently issue it in such a piecemeal way.

Most assistive technology-related services operate completely separately and independently from one another, resulting in duplication, poor use of resources, and wastage, not to mention the effect on the service user of having to undergo multiple assessments.

One of the results of failing to provide assistive technologies and disability equipment effectively is significant unnecessary cost for the health and care economy, for example through delayed hospital discharges, and unnecessary hospital and care home admissions. Providing services inappropriately is always a false economy.

Incorporating assistive technologies into the delivery of health and care provision is a whole-systems responsibility. It starts with good planning, commissioning and governance. This inevitably flows through to good service provision and clinical involvement. Each of these service areas needs to be clear about their respective responsibilities. There also need to be measurable outcomes and standards in place.

This Code of Practice is designed to address this, and offers a template for commissioning and providing services; it includes clearly defined and specific standards and measurable outcomes.

Following the Code, in all its parts, will go a long way in overcoming many of the difficulties highlighted above and will significantly improve both clinical and financial outcomes. It will also help to identify where weaknesses are within the whole system and allow root causes to be traced. Following the Code will also enable any equipment-related strategies to be achieved.

The Code, in some or all its parts, relates mainly to disability equipment, wheelchair and seating services. It also applies more generally to other assistive technology-related services; there are certain Code Standards which provide a link to related services, which will assist with integration and offering seamless provision.

PART ONE

COMMISSIONING AND GOVERNANCE

Introduction to Code Standards 1 to 8

The importance of commissioning and planning equipment and wheelchair services should not be underestimated. Whilst safe and effective equipment provision is the result of whole-system efforts, designing and commissioning services appropriately is crucial to meeting service users' needs and achieving the right outcomes. Should this part of the process be wrong, with inadequate funding and unclear specifications, then a poor level of overall service will inevitably ensue.

Commissioners should understand what it is they want to commission, be clear about what the provider's responsibilities are, and have the right clinical and technical skills and resources to achieve their aims.

Generally speaking, equipment providers will only respond to the requirements set out in the service specification. This means it is important for commissioners to understand what it is they are trying to achieve, what service users' needs are, and how they can be met.

Commissioners also need to be aware of the underlying demand for these services, including anticipated growth and unmet need.

It is equally important to have systems in place to ensure what is being specified by the commissioners is actually being delivered by the provider, and thus the desired outcome is being achieved. Therefore, good governance, procurement and contract management arrangements for the provision of equipment services are crucial.

In some cases, poor service levels and quality can be owing to the absence of relevant data and information in the service specification and contract. Underestimation of demand can ultimately result in services costing more than originally anticipated. Specifying service requirements poorly can also significantly impact upon other care-related organisations and services, and can affect long-term partnership working, for example.

Ensuring the provider has sufficient data and information has to be balanced against being too specific about what the provider should do, and how they should do it, as this can sometimes stifle innovation and ties services into always being delivered the same way. It is best to develop clear and measurable outcomes, supported by activity data.

There is no doubt that it is a difficult task for commissioners to understand and plan for both current and future equipment needs and demands, whilst managing expectations and the limitations of their organisations, as well as being constrained by the lack of wider partnership and joined-up working opportunities with other related agencies; they may also be working within restricted eligibility criteria, with limited funding. There needs to be dialogue with public health partners to understand the underlying need, and establishing good relationships with wider partners enables mutual benefits to be identified and realised. This needs to be supported by having meaningful data and information, and robust reporting arrangements, regarding performance.

There is a real danger when commissioning equipment-related services in isolation, without joined-up working with partner agencies, that whilst the immediate clinical (health) need of the service user is met, in their daily lives they experience difficulties because their wider needs have not been considered, e.g. they can't use their equipment in different settings and environments. A silo mentality is short-term and counter-productive as it shifts additional responsibility and cost onto other agencies, as well as being burdensome for the service user. Joined-up working is essential to avoid duplication and cost for public sector agencies and to improve user experience.

Despite the abundance of health and safety-related legislation, there have been numerous incidents involving unsafe supply or use of equipment, often avoidable had the provider acted appropriately. When specifying service requirements, it is not advisable to use general statements about legal and welfare obligations, e.g. 'the provider must comply with all relevant health and safety requirements'. It is important for commissioners to specify in detail the actual legal and welfare-related obligations the provider is expected to comply with, as it is all too easy for assumptions to be made about what service providers should be doing; providers need to be made aware of these expectations to ensure they have allocated sufficient resources to meeting requirements.

Appendix 1 outlines some of the main legislation which directly applies to the commissioning and provision of equipment. Each of these places a significant responsibility, and in some cases a duty, upon commissioners (and providers), and all can have serious consequences, if breached.

It is good practice for commissioners to make service users aware of the level of service to expect as it can be disappointing at the end of a long wait to be told they cannot receive a particular service or product. Information about services provided and entitlement could be in the form of a patients' charter, or a visual representation of the care pathway, in accordance with the service model.

CODE STANDARD 1

Service Requirements and Specifications

OUTCOME
The requirements, expectations and aims for the delivery of an equipment service are clearly specified and communicated, realistic, and easy to be interpreted and understood.

Introduction to Code Standard 1

Without the equipment provider having a clear understanding about what it is they are expected by the commissioners to do, in terms of service requirements, aims and outcomes, it is very likely that problems will arise.

Clearly specifying service expectations and standards, and having the right controls and measures in place for ensuring compliance, are key in the delivery of an all-round successful equipment service.

Where there is little data regarding activity, or where a new service is being commissioned, it is wise for the commissioner and provider to work hand in hand and to be flexible, so that activity levels and funding can be readjusted retrospectively where necessary. Otherwise problems may persist throughout the duration of the contract if activity levels prove inaccurate.

It is important for providers, service users and carers to know what the aims and principles of the service are, and what level of service they can expect to receive.

1.1 Service requirements, aims and principles have been clearly specified, in the form of a service level agreement, service specification and/or a contract, as appropriate.

1.2 A realistic expectation of activity levels, including approximate numbers for each type of activity, together with agreed tolerances, etc., have been clearly specified. The contractual agreement specifies the procedure to be taken should activity levels exceed or fall below these tolerances.

1.3 Current and future demands on services over the duration of the contract have been considered, factoring in any expected growth in demand where, for example, the number of service users rises owing to the increasing average age of the population.

1.4 Allowance has been made for any anticipated changes in equipment design, and new developments which could arise over the duration of the contract.

1.5 Prior to commencing the contract, there has been dialogue with the provider to ensure that the requirements and expectations placed upon the provider are realistic, and budget allocations have been arrived at using an appropriate calculated formula. Where there is no historic or suitable data available to form such an agreement, i.e. when a completely new service is being set up, frequent reviews are agreed with the provider to monitor and assess the level of activities.

1.6 Allowance has been made for the costs of compliance for the provider to meet all the requirements as set out in the specification and/or contract.

1.7 General or vague statements have not been used within the service specification and/or contract, etc. where ambiguity could be to the detriment of service provision. For example, requesting that the provider complies with all relevant health and safety requirements is too broad, and could be misleading. Providers should be given a comprehensive list setting out actual requirements and obligations, e.g. 'a portable appliance test is carried out on all portable electrical appliances in accordance with the Electricity at Work Regulations

1989.' (Note the costs of compliance with the cited legislation will also need to be considered.)

1.8 Service level agreements/service specifications and/or contracts are reviewed at fixed intervals, e.g. annually, and reviews involve suitable stakeholders and users of the services.

1.9 There is a patients' charter, or similar information package, outlining the levels of service which users can expect to receive, and types of need that will be met, e.g. short or long-term, or occasional use.

1.10 There is a visual representation of the care pathway available, in accordance with the service model. The care pathway must reflect all key stages of the service as specified in the service description and ensure maximum response times for each stage of the pathway are set. This is communicated to all interested and relevant parties, e.g. service user, General Practitioners.

1.11 There is a list of the equipment types that are provided under statutory provision; this includes both simple and complex equipment. Any approved third-party providers or suppliers also have access to this list.

1.12 Roles, responsibilities and accountabilities of the commissioners, providers and any third-party providers or suppliers, are clearly specified.

1.13 Where different parts of the service are provided by different providers, e.g. routine and complex equipment, and maintenance, this is clearly specified in corresponding contracts and/or agreements.

1.14 There is a requirement for service providers to submit proper clinical audit and clinical effectiveness reviews. Particular attention should be paid to service user satisfaction, with an emphasis on needs being met.

1.15 Providers are actively encouraged to suggest and use innovative ways to deliver the service, taking advantage of the range of technology available.

CODE STANDARD 2

Partnerships and Joint Working Arrangements

OUTCOME

Sector-wide integrated commissioning and joint working is in place, together with joint funding arrangements (where appropriate) with all relevant agencies, to ensure duplication and inefficiency are minimised, and to make sure all the needs of the service user can be met in a coordinated and timely manner.

Introduction to Code Standard 2

There are many statutory organisations funding delivery of similar equipment-related services, e.g. health, local authority (housing, education and social care).

In view of the scope for duplication, time delays and inefficiencies when providing entirely separate services for the same service user, efforts have been made over recent years to improve integration and joint working between relevant organisations.

Commissioning arrangements should include plans for multi-agency and joined-up working to ensure the totality of users' needs are met as seamlessly and effortlessly as possible. This will require liaison arrangements with, for example, the housing service for adaptations, the education department for special needs, and other equipment-related services, including prosthetics, orthotics, telecare and community equipment services.

Simply including in service specifications that providers, including clinical staff, should work in a joined-up and integrated manner, is not sufficient to ensure this actually happens in practice. These ambitions need to be firstly established and agreed at a commissioning level, for them to be effective.

There are many voluntary and private sector organisations, and wider support services, such as housing agencies, providing equipment-related functions. As yet the benefits of these organisations and sectors fully engaging in joint working for achieving seamless, timely and cost effective equipment supply have not been fully explored and realised. We are living in an era when these opportunities should be embraced.

2.1 There are formal agreements in place for funding integrated commissioning and joint delivery of services between relevant agencies responsible for arranging equipment services locally.

2.2 Interdependencies with relevant organisations, services and departments are listed, and formal links are established with these, to assist with referrals and to ensure the service user has a clear pathway for accessing services, and can be signposted and navigated between services effortlessly.

2.3 Measures are in place to support service users during critical life-change transitions, e.g. child to adult service user, loss of key carer (e.g. parent), university to workplace, including jointly commissioned and/or integrated services.

2.4 Where appropriate, there are multi-agency or integration protocols to ensure the assessment and provision of equipment meets all the service user's needs, and allows for services to be provided promptly as soon as a need has been identified.

2.5 The available partnership and joint working agreements include (but are not limited to):

- names of statutory partners
- purpose of the agreement

- date and duration of agreement
- which Health Act flexibilities apply (if applicable)
- the aims, outcomes and targets set by the partnership or commissioning body
- who the service users are/who the service is for. This is defined in terms of service user group, age range, LA, NHS and partner areas, etc.
- how the services are to be accessed, e.g. assessment and eligibility
- how much resource is to be committed to the partnership by each commissioning partner and any organisational services in support of the partnership, e.g. information, premises, procurement support
- how resource levels are updated, especially the budget-building exercise for future years
- how the agreement is managed, e.g. joint governance group to set annual plans and targets, monitor performance, agree variations, manage reviews/renewal, and reporting to others
- when the agreement is subject to review, and frequency of reviews
- how performance is measured.

2.6 There is evidence of good working relationships between the different organisations and sectors involved in the provision of equipment. This includes other arrangements outside of formal partnerships and joint working, e.g. links with acute hospitals and third-sector organisations.

2.7 Where there are gaps in provision, unmet needs or non-provision in certain areas, alternative methods of provision are in place, including, for example, partnerships and strategic alliances with third-sector organisations.

2.8 Partnerships or joint working arrangements are able to offer transparent evidence of their processes for coordination of service provision that reflects a person-centred approach to meeting people's 'whole-life' needs.

2.9 Alternative funding options, e.g. direct payments, personal health budgets, vouchers (for wheelchairs), are considered in the planning phase, and arrangements for support when obtaining local personalised services. These initiatives are not inhibited by partnerships or joint working arrangements for equipment.

CODE STANDARD 3

Funding Arrangements

> **OUTCOME**
> Services are adequately funded in relation to requirements and expectations.

Introduction to Code Standard 3

Funding for equipment services can be problematic; this is often due to the relationship between activity and cost not being fully understood. If services are inappropriately funded, significant problems can arise for the provider of services, and can result in dangerous and even illegal practice. This is especially true where services have to take 'shortcuts' in service standards, in order to operate within the funds allocated to them. Not only can inappropriate funding cause risks to arise, it may cost the wider health and care economy more in the longer term by having to fund more costly episodes of care, e.g. more people being admitted to hospitals and care homes, and people developing pressure sores.

Over the duration of certain equipment contracts, activity will rise significantly because of the increasing average age of the population. It is important, therefore, that both current and future funding is considered.

Furthermore, in an era of choice and control, it is important that alternative funding options are considered and made available to service users and/or their carers, as another means of obtaining equipment. The funding of this would have to be carefully planned and managed.

3.1 Service providers are appropriately funded to enable them to meet the requirements of their service specifications, for the duration of the contract, and to meet any policy and regulatory requirements.

3.2 There are clear and agreed activity tolerance levels providers are expected to operate within.

3.3 There is a clear formula in place demonstrating how funding allocations have been calculated; an impact assessment is provided in the case where equipment provision is not adequately funded, or if funding is withdrawn.

3.4 Funding allocations are not based entirely upon previous budgets and/or spend, but match what the provider is actually being asked to undertake for the relevant period. Retrospective funding may be necessary in some instances, where, for example, a new service has been set up, i.e. in the absence of sufficient data to allocate funds, funding can be allocated after running the service for an agreed period.

3.5 A schedule is available showing a breakdown of activities and related costs, e.g. deliveries, collections, maintenance. A breakdown of expenditure for different elements of equipment is also available, e.g. complex and children's equipment.

3.6 Where relevant, expenditure breakdown also covers third-party provider and supplier activity.

3.7 Where appropriate, funding includes whole-life costs for equipment, e.g. maintenance, replacement parts.

3.8 Where alternative funding options for equipment are offered, e.g. personal budgets, personal health budgets or vouchers (for wheelchairs), there is clarity over whole-life costs, i.e. who is responsible for paying maintenance and replacing broken parts, and ongoing support.

3.9 Equipment providers have been actively involved in providing costs for the running of operations. This may be through the submission of a pre-purchase questionnaire, tender submissions, or similar mechanism. Where in-house services are contracted to provide a service, an exercise to consider the costs of compliance with the service specification has been undertaken; this is to ensure demands on the provider are realistic within the funds allocated.

3.10 Expenditure on all specific categories of equipment is monitored whether or not equipment is integrated or pooled. This also includes a breakdown of amounts paid via alternative funding routes, e.g. direct payments, personal budgets, vouchers, or to third-party providers or suppliers.

3.11 Financial allocations for equipment services relate to needs within the population and are developed as part of any joint health and social care strategic planning – this may include other partners.

3.12 Funding is made available to support Continuing Professional Development, education and training of all staff working within the service. This may include both in-house and external courses and should, as a matter of course, involve training on the features and benefits of equipment on the service's agreed range, as well as support to identify new and emerging products and technologies.

CODE STANDARD 4

Contractual Arrangements

> **OUTCOME**
> Equipment provision is subject to formal contracting arrangements, and documentation is in place which has clear terms and conditions, with roles and responsibilities specified. This includes a clear service specification.

Introduction to Code Standard 4

In the past there have been cases where equipment services have been provided without formal contractual arrangements being in place, or using old and outdated specifications bearing no relation to current demands and activity; this is usually owing to services being in-house and having evolved over the years.

Without formal contractual arrangements in place, service providers will find it difficult to deliver an efficient and effective service.

It is important where several contracts are in place to cover different aspects of the service, e.g. external suppliers or therapists, that there is harmony between them, and a shared outcome.

4.1 Services are provided under a formal signed contract, in the case of an external provider, or an internal Service Level Agreement (SLA) for non-contracted-out services.

4.2 Contracts enable the provider to integrate and collaborate, where necessary, with other relevant agencies and services to ensure all the equipment-related needs of the service user can be met in a coordinated and timely way.

4.3 Where there is integrated or partnership provision, this is in evidence by a formal partnership agreement.

4.4 Where there are several independent providers, commissioned to provide different parts of the full service, they can demonstrate cooperation between each other and across the service user pathway.

4.5 Roles and responsibilities for each of the respective organisations, and key individuals involved, have been clearly set out within formal documentation.

4.6 There is flexibility within the contractual arrangements to enable alterations and changes to be made throughout the contract period, to allow for changes in policy, demand, or advancements in equipment technology, for example.

4.7 Contracts and/or formal agreements carry local legal endorsement.

CODE STANDARD 5

Legal, Regulatory and Welfare Obligations

> **OUTCOME**
> The legal, regulatory and welfare requirements, including individual and organisational duties and responsibilities, relating to the provision of equipment services, are carefully considered, clearly documented and communicated.

Introduction to Code Standard 5

The legal, regulatory and welfare duties, obligations and parameters for the provision of equipment services are extensive, ranging from various UN Conventions, e.g. Rights of Disabled People, Rights of the Child; criminal, health and safety, medical device, welfare-related and consumer protection laws, standards and regulations. These are in place to protect the service user, staff and organisations alike. Duties and obligations could unknowingly be breached without appropriate measures in place to ensure compliance.

It is very important for commissioners, providers, clinical professionals and service users to be clear about the particular legal, regulatory and welfare-related duties and obligations that pertain to them; otherwise assumptions could be made about who is responsible, which sometimes results in gaps in provision and significant breaches.

In an era of offering choice, together with the growing demand for personal budgets, and other alternative means of obtaining equipment, e.g. vouchers for wheelchairs, it is important that the legal implications are considered.

5.1 The legal, regulatory and welfare-related boundaries that equipment providers are expected to operate within, and in some case report on, are clearly identified and written into all Memoranda of Understanding, service level agreements, service specifications, contract agreements, and/or partnership agreements, as appropriate.

5.2 Information relating to legal, regulatory and welfare obligations is communicated effectively, and in appropriate formats, to all responsible individuals and organisations highlighting their specific responsibilities.

5.3 Information is available to service users setting out their legal entitlement to assessments and equipment, together with (regulatory) standards the provider organisation is working to. This may be in the form of a patients' charter, for example.

Author's note

Although subject to change, examples of health and safety and consumer protection legislation pertinent to these services are set out in Appendix 1. The legislation provided is relevant at the time of writing this Code of Practice; it is not exhaustive and is only intended to be a general guide. Organisations are advised to seek the advice of health and safety and legal departments within their own organisation.

Note that health and welfare-related legislation and specific regulatory obligations have not been included in this Code as these are subject to regular change, and are sometimes different across the countries of the UK. Please, therefore, keep yourself up to date with current legislation and regulatory obligations applicable in the country you work in.

CODE STANDARD 6

Governance and Risk Management

> **OUTCOME**
> Clear and comprehensive governance and risk management strategies exist, covering all aspects of service delivery, whilst ensuring appropriate reporting mechanisms and controls are in place for monitoring purposes.

Introduction to Code Standard 6

Equipment services are generally commissioned and governed by health and/or local authorities. Often there are partnership boards or joint commissioning or management arrangements in place.

Where partnership or joint working arrangements are not in place, it can be problematic to maintain high standards of governance and risk management when, for example, one authority commissions a service, and has governance and risk management responsibilities for it, but the service itself, and the service users, have interfaces with other related agencies beyond the control of the original commissioner. There needs to be strong governance, and risk management links between the different agencies.

The commissioning and governance responsibilities with regards to equipment provision are very broad. Responsibilities include, for example: ensuring all risk issues are managed appropriately; compliance with legislation, quality, performance, finances, contractual arrangements and clinical governance. Without the presence of a formal governance structure, service provision could become ineffective, inefficient, unsafe, and even illegal.

Commissioners are also responsible for making sure the needs of the service user are met and that the governance of procured services reflects how service user rights are protected.

It is sometimes assumed that outsourcing certain components of service provision reduces or removes statutory responsibility and accountability, especially for governance and risk management arrangements. However, commissioners should be clear that in these instances they retain the responsibility to ensure governance and risk issues are assessed, managed, communicated and monitored.

6.1 Governance structures and arrangements are in place and are clearly documented. The documentation outlines specific areas of responsibility, together with monitoring procedures and named individuals/posts responsible for ensuring procedures are followed.

6.2 Governance and risk management arrangements form part of all contractual arrangements.

6.3 Decisions, and the process for making decisions, with regards to governance issues, are transparent and involve relevant stakeholders, including service users.

6.4 A risk management strategy exists and includes, but is not limited to, such things as:

- roles and responsibilities of commissioners and providers
- links to other risk-related services, groups and boards, e.g. Medical Device Management Board
- medical device management
- health and safety and risk management
- accreditation process of third-party contractors
- exit strategy if the provider can no longer provide a service.

6.5 There is a service-specific, care-related, risk management strategy in place which addresses, for example, the accessibility of services, the care pathway, prevention of deterioration of conditions and risk to carers, and management of care to service users. This is clearly documented, communicated and understood by all relevant parties.

6.6 Where formal partnership or joint working arrangements exist, these incorporate a governance, risk management and risk sharing section, specifying processes for identifying and responding to risks, alongside partner roles and responsibilities. A section relating to management of financial risk is also included.

6.7 A designated and named lead has been appointed with overall responsibility for medical device management relating to the provision of equipment.

6.8 The complaints procedure is transparent and easily accessible to people with differing communication needs; advocacy is available where necessary. It separates areas of responsibility and clearly sets out contact details and processes for different aspects of the service.

CODE STANDARD 7

Eligibility Criteria

> **OUTCOME**
> There is clarity over eligibility criteria, fairness and consistency in their use and application.

Introduction to Code Standard 7

Many problems can stem from inappropriate eligibility criteria, e.g. difficulty managing demand and finances, and service users not having their needs met satisfactorily. These problems are often compounded when financial resources for both the NHS and local authorities come under pressure.

Changes in central government policy can also influence the eligibility criteria applied.

Despite the difficulties, it is vital that there is clarity around what level of service people can expect and will receive, and that this is properly communicated. It is equally important for people to be made aware of needs that will 'not' be met, e.g. short-term needs. This may be in the form of setting out 'exclusions'. This helps to manage expectations and avoid disappointment.

Eligibility criteria should be very clear and easy to interpret and understand, allowing decisions to be made relatively easily. It should be flexible enough to allow for changes and developments in equipment design and advances in technology, and also for innovative solutions to meet particular needs. Special circumstances should also be accommodated to allow for people with rapidly progressing conditions and short life expectancy, for example.

Eligibility criteria should also have scope to allow for joint working and funding with relevant stakeholders to ensure holistic needs can be met.

7.1 The decision-making process used for equipment provision is based entirely upon, and in accordance with the eligibility criteria. This factors in and considers the service user outcomes, e.g. what is the consequence of not providing equipment.

7.2 Eligibility criteria and supporting guidance are not so limiting, that as a result only one part of the service user's needs are met. Wider issues are considered, such as, for example, the complexity of conditions, e.g. rapidly progressing conditions, anticipatory needs, special assessments, pressure and posture needs, and accessories.

7.3 It is very clear from the eligibility criteria used, what needs will and will not be met, together with the justification and rationale for these decisions.

7.4 Eligibility criteria are not so rigid and inflexible that people in special circumstances cannot access the service, or that the wider needs of the service user cannot be met.

7.5 Eligibility criteria reflect that the assessment and provision of equipment is based on an individual's needs, and is not used as a means of rationing/containing costs.

7.6 It is clearly set out in guidance, or a patients' charter, a 'core offer' stating what will be provided as a minimum and the needs that will be met.

7.7 The eligibility criteria and supporting guidance used for deciding on equipment provision is documented and communicated to all relevant individuals involved in issuing equipment, and service users, if requested.

7.8   Where relevant, provision of help and advice is available to people who fall outside the stated eligibility criteria and who would benefit from purchasing equipment privately, or by using alternative funding options, e.g. a direct payment, personal health budget or voucher (for wheelchairs).

7.9   Where organisations or services have come together by a formal partnership or joint working arrangement and developed single, or shared, eligibility criteria, this is publicly available for all staff and service users. Details of eligibility criteria are included in any agreements.

7.10 Where alternative funding options are offered for equipment, e.g. direct payment or voucher, these are supported by eligibility criteria.

7.11 Eligibility criteria consider the different settings and environments where equipment is likely to be used, e.g. nursing or residential homes, and reflect the realistic aspirations of the service user, considering where the service user may want to or need to use the equipment in the near future.

CODE STANDARD 8

Contract and Performance Management

> **OUTCOME**
> Contracts are appropriately managed and reviewed to ensure performance is optimal, and this is evidenced sufficiently to meet audit requirements.

Introduction to Code Standard 8

Contract and performance management involves systematically and efficiently managing the creation of the contract, its execution and analysis. This serves to maximise operational and financial performance and minimise risk.

There is an assumption that good contract and performance management begins with post-award activities. Whilst this is true in part, successful contract and performance management is most effective if pre-award activities are properly carried out, e.g. due diligence on potential suppliers, development of good performance measures to include in the service specification.

Management of contracts with service providers is an area that can be easily overlooked or taken for granted. Without effective contract management arrangements in place it is almost certain that good performance standards will be lacking. Contract management responsibilities should be assigned to named individuals or roles, in order to keep a close rein on all the different aspects of the service.

It is important that robust and meaningful indicators, standards and measurable outcomes are used to capture and ascertain performance levels; there are many performance indicators available to support this. It is equally important to ensure that the means for collecting the data are robust, e.g. IT systems, especially where audit is concerned.

It is also important that contract management is proactive and responsive to ensure that any issues with performance, or changes in activity, can be identified and addressed in a timely way.

Where authorities use third-party providers or suppliers, it is also important to ensure that relevant performance-related issues can be captured.

Whilst it is ultimately the responsibility of the commissioner to ensure the contract is being executed properly and that performance is optimal, there is also a significant onus on the service provider to monitor and self-regulate their own compliance against the requirements of the contract and other relevant performance and quality standards.

Where appropriate, the provider should be encouraged to use self-regulation and reporting tools as this can ease the administrative burden on the commissioner and provider alike, and will help to proactively manage all aspects of contract and performance management.

8.1   There are robust contract and performance management measures in place for ensuring optimum contract performance is achieved, which also reflect service user satisfaction. The table in Appendix 2 sets out a guide to some of the more general contract management indicators that can be used for measuring certain aspects of performance. Other local measures can be used in addition.

8.2   Clearly defined, realistic and measurable standards and outcomes have been set for the provider to work toward, and these are reported on in a timely and consistent way.

8.3   Contract performance data is obtained from the provider, including reliable management reports and clinical audit, where relevant, and this data is reviewed and analysed appropriately.

8.4 In order to ensure contracts are appropriately managed, there is a designated lead individual/role with overall contract management responsibilities.

8.5 There is flexibility and scope within contractual arrangements to allow for any future increases in activity or where new developments in equipment become available, for example.

8.6 Performance is ascertained by various methods, for example, relevant key performance indicators (KPIs), reporting against defined outcomes and service aims, contract management tools, relevant quality measures and feedback from service users. Local measures and indicators may also be in place.

8.7 Management information includes, but is not limited to, referral data, service user numbers and profiles, assessments, waiting times, unmet needs and third-party providers and suppliers.

8.8 The performance measures in place satisfy pertinent audit and inspection purposes, in terms of data collection processes, validation, robustness, relevance and accuracy.

8.9 Relevant contract and performance data is captured electronically from internal IT systems, as manual collection of data will not generally meet auditors' requirements.

8.10 Locally defined, realistic and measurable outcomes have been developed for the provider to work towards and report on.

8.11 Where applicable, contract and performance management ascertains the reasons for failure to achieve agreed levels of performance and outcomes, and the potential impact (if known).

8.12 Regardless of the number of providers and third-party contractors supplying different aspects of service delivery, management reports are available to demonstrate individual and collective performance, so an overall assessment of service provision can be made.

8.13 Where an arrangement is set up with third-party providers or suppliers, there is a written, and mutually agreed, understanding about performance and contractual obligations.

8.14 Where equipment and services are provided via alternative funding options, e.g. direct payment, a personal health budget, voucher (for wheelchairs), feedback is sought formally from service users to ascertain their experience as a matter of course.

8.15 Service providers are encouraged to have suitable systems/tools in place to monitor and self-regulate their own compliance against the requirements of the contract and other relevant quality, safety and performance standards.

8.16 There is a nominated individual with governance responsibility for ensuring the providing organisation's IT systems, and the information provided by the systems, are robust.

PART TWO

SERVICE

PROVISION

Introduction to Code Standards 9 to 23

This part of the Code particularly focuses on the operational and stores functions of service provision.

Operational aspects of the provision of equipment include providing a stores facility, procurement, logistics, delivery and collection of equipment, decontamination and maintenance, equipment installation and demonstrations. Very often equipment providers are required to support a range of stakeholders, with many expectations and obligations to fulfil.

Equipment providers offer a critical service, which if not provided safely or effectively, can put the lives and wellbeing of service users at risk. Poor service provision can also have a knock-on effect upon wider health and care-related services, e.g. through unnecessary hospital admissions. It is therefore crucial that equipment providers are properly resourced and equipped in order to meet the demands and expectations placed upon them.

In addition to operational aspects, providers are expected to abide by many legal, health and safety and medical device management duties and obligations. It is essential that providers are aware of these and that there is assurance of their ability to comply with these.

Where alternative funding options are offered as a way for service users to obtain equipment, e.g. direct payments, personal health budgets or vouchers (for wheelchairs), it is important that there is clarity for the provider, where appropriate, around ongoing specific roles and responsibilities, particularly in relation to product safety, maintenance, complaints and liability issues.

The use of third-party contractors for some parts of service provision does not remove the legal responsibilities of statutory providers and commissioners. Should parts of equipment provision be outsourced, e.g. decontamination, by the main provider, then there is a responsibility on the main provider to ensure legal obligations are met.

This part of the Code of Practice is applicable equally to outsourced service providers and to in-house public sector providers. Appendix 1 lists some of the main health and safety and consumer protection legislation relating to the provision of equipment.

CODE STANDARD 9

Operational Management

> **OUTCOME**
> All operational and contract management responsibilities are clearly defined with designated leads.

Introduction to Code Standard 9

In an equipment store, operational management responsibilities are very broad and cover almost all aspects of service delivery. Most services will have a single operational manager, or contracts manager (particularly for outsourced services), with ultimate responsibility for ensuring all aspects of operational management are achieved. There may also be other managers with particular responsibilities, e.g. technical manager, but this will very much depend on the size and scope of the service.

9.1   The operational lead, or contract manager, is supported by an operational team and ensures, has knowledge of, and is able to demonstrate how the following aspects of service delivery are being achieved:

i   Financial management
Budget management; pooled funding (where appropriate); invoicing, etc.

ii   Service management
Strategy of service; management of projects.

iii Performance and information management

Production of performance statistics; identifying trends and projections; issue of data reports.

iv Information management

Management of all information technologies, including setup and scheduling of reports; ensuring information is accurate.

v Stock management

Product management; managing trends; maintaining safety stock levels; ensuring equipment recall systems exist; monitoring and updating IT systems; management of satellite (buffer) stores (where appropriate).

vi Store management

Building management, including all satellite stores; facilities management.

vii Staff management

Staff training; handling staff-related issues; ensuring appropriate staffing levels are available; criminal record checks.

viii Contract management

Monitoring performance; monitoring third-party supplier performance; writing contracts and service level agreements with third-party providers.

ix Logistics management

Vehicle and fleet management; managing urgent and out-of-hours deliveries.

x Procurement management

Facilitating equipment selection processes; carrying out negotiations with suppliers; developing product selection specifications.

xi Asset management

Managing planned maintenance, repair, recycling, refurbishment, scrapping or writing off, and traceability of all assets.

xii Health and safety and risk management

Management of all health and safety and risk issues through formal policies, procedures, assessments, and monitoring arrangements, where appropriate. Example areas will include: maintenance of all equipment, medical device management.

xiii Clinical services interface

Meeting clinical need; addressing clinical priorities; prescriber training.

xiv Customer service/patient care

Dealing with customer satisfaction, complaints, and having a formal complaints procedure; having a contact number and individual to handle customer issues.

xv Quality management

Having Total Quality Management (TQM) systems in place; carrying out regular 'spot checks', and regular audits.

xvi Policies and procedures

Writing and updating policies; implementing new policies; having processes in place for ensuring policies and procedures are being followed.

CODE STANDARD 10

Quality Management Systems

OUTCOME

Quality management systems are built into the service provider's business practice.

Introduction to Code Standard 10

Given the nature of equipment provision, in that services are generally delivered to vulnerable people, it is most important that a good quality service is provided.

Quality is not something that happens of its own accord, it has to be properly managed. There are various approved techniques and standards available for managing quality, e.g. ISO 9001:2008, otherwise known as quality management systems. Quality management is considered to have three main components: *quality control*, *quality assurance* and *quality improvement*. Quality management is focused not only on product quality, but also the means to achieve it. Quality management therefore uses quality assurance and control of processes as well as products to achieve more consistent quality.

In an environment where equipment is provided, examples of quality management might be something as simple as having a procedure for testing new products, or a guide for assembling equipment. Quality will be consistent throughout all aspects of the service, ranging from procurement processes to decontamination and storage standards.

10.1 A robust quality management system is in place which covers all operational aspects of service delivery; this will be a recognised British, European, Harmonised, e.g. BS/EN, or ideally, International Standard, e.g. ISO 9001:2008, or equivalent. The requirements that a good quality management system will aim to cover include, but are not limited to:

- a set of procedures that cover all key processes, e.g. operational policy
- monitoring of processes to ensure they are effective
- keeping adequate records
- checking output for defects, with appropriate and corrective action where necessary
- regularly reviewing individual processes and the quality system itself for effectiveness
- facilitating continual improvement.

10.2 There are documented and up-to-date policies and procedures in place, accessible to all staff members, covering all operational functions of the service.

10.3 All staff are fully aware of, and are working to, the relevant section of the policies and procedures applicable to their role.

CODE STANDARD 11

Training and Qualifications

> **OUTCOME**
> Operational and technical staff are appropriately trained and qualified in relation to the tasks they are required to undertake.

Introduction to Code Standard 11

This particular Code Standard pertains more to operational and technical staff, and not clinical staff, as it covers general aspects relating to provision of equipment. Training regarding the clinical aspect is addressed in more detail in Code Standard 27.

Training is an area often overlooked where the provision of equipment is concerned. Training needs to be viewed as broadly as possible, covering all aspects of service provision, e.g. stores management, technical skills, etc. The Medicines and Healthcare Products Regulatory Agency (MHRA) has emphasised the importance of appropriate training in its 2006 *Managing Medical Devices* guidance for healthcare and social services organisations DB2006 (05), and has detailed the considerations to be given for each role. The guidance states that all aspects of training in relation to service provision should be incorporated into a policy, or procedures, document.

Training issues are also important where third-party providers or suppliers are used; in particular, training should be considered in relation to demonstration, fitting and installation of equipment.

Training, with regards to equipment, needs to be viewed from three different perspectives:

i   management of equipment provision
ii technical skills
iii clinical and professional users (qualifications and training for clinical and professional staff are dealt with in more detail in Code Standard 27)

11.1 All training-related policies and procedures are incorporated into a policy document, and are accessible and communicated to all members of staff.

11.2 Where service providers use third-party providers and suppliers, they have specified that their staff have to be adequately trained.

11.3 Depending on their role in equipment provision, all staff are suitably trained and qualified in some or all of the following subjects:

- policy and procedures – local, corporate and national
- health, safety and legislation
- health and safety management (for management)
- performance and contract management
- stores and stock management
- technical and maintenance management
- equipment IT systems – store, clinical and information
- financial management, including pooled and joint funding arrangements
- customer care (relevant where there is service user interface).

11.4 Staff employed to undertake complex and specialist repair and maintenance responsibilities are competent to do so, depending upon the level of technical work required. Where appropriate, there are training contracts in place with suppliers/manufacturers to train on technically complex equipment and new technologies.

Note

As an example, the organisation Semta has developed occupational standards specifically for equipment technicians, with levels 2 and 3. Semta is the Sector Skills Council for science, engineering and manufacturing technologies in the UK. Examples of some duties carried out at the different levels as set out by Semta can be viewed as supporting guidance in Appendix 3.

Rehabilitation engineers (or equivalent) should be formally qualified to degree level or equivalent, and may be working toward State Registration as a clinical technologist through the Institute of Physics and Engineering in Medicine (www.ipem.ac.uk/). Training competencies and standards for clinical engineers, rehabilitation engineers and other healthcare science professionals are available on the RESMaG (www.resmag.org.uk) and National Wheelchair Managers Forum (www.wheelchairmanagers.nhs.uk/) websites.

11.5 Where applicable, staff coming into contact with the public are trained in appropriate communication methods, including communication tactics with deaf and hard of hearing people, or people with visual impairments, for example. Where appropriate, consideration for language is given.

11.6 Where staff come into direct contact with service users, they are provided with appropriate awareness training, looking at the qualities needed to work with people with disabilities.

11.7 Training is provided to staff by accredited or approved trainers.

11.8 Ongoing and refresher training is available to reflect the developments in the range of equipment and changes in technical specification.

CODE STANDARD 12

Information Technology and Information Management

> **OUTCOME**
> Information is meaningful, produced in a timely manner and suitable format, and managed and communicated appropriately.

Introduction to Code Standard 12

The success of equipment provision, from an overall performance perspective, is partly dependent upon the robustness and quality of the data provided by the equipment provider's IT systems. A good specialist IT system is the backbone of service provision, and should be able to produce good quality information.

There are a variety of IT systems available to help manage the operational aspects of the service and to monitor and self-regulate compliance against quality, safety and performance standards. Investment in such systems offers a range of benefits in terms of making services more efficient and effective, and significantly reducing the administrative burden of having to capture information manually.

It is helpful to commissioners of services if they are provided with robust and meaningful data relating to activity and trends, for example, to enable them to make informed and conscious decisions about the equipment service, which in turn could lead to further investment.

Agreeing information reporting requirements at the start of a contract is important for maintaining good working relationships with commissioners and those procuring the service, and failure to do so can allow misunderstandings to arise, which puts a strain on relationships as well as impairing performance.

It is important to ensure that those operating the IT systems understand their functionalities, and are appropriately trained, on an ongoing basis, to use them. To ensure information and data are accurate, and that high standards of accuracy are maintained, it is essential that regular data quality checks are in place.

IT systems are also crucial for collecting referral and clinical information. They can also provide a virtual authorisation check, and can offer virtual budget management solutions for budget holders.

12.1 IT systems are 'fit for purpose', meeting all clinical, financial and operational functionality requirements, whilst adhering to local and national data protection issues.

12.2 IT systems can generate all necessary performance-related reports, with the ability to drill down information, as appropriate.

12.3 Suitable IT systems/tools are in place to monitor and self-regulate compliance against the requirements of the contract and other relevant quality, safety and performance standards and outcomes.

12.4 There is evidence of audit and governance ('policing') arrangements in place to ensure the information provided by third-party sources to the IT systems is accurate, and also that the data provided is being input correctly; this is supported by procedures. Audit and data quality checks take place on a regular basis.

12.5 IT systems used for the provision of equipment have the ability to identify the location of equipment in the event of a recall.

12.6 Training in the use of the various IT systems used within equipment services is delivered by someone competent to do so.

12.7 Training is provided to all members of staff using the systems, and peripheral technologies, e.g. hand-held devices. This includes: management; stores operatives; administrators; technicians; drivers; prescribers.

12.8 Appropriate certification with renewal dates is issued with initial training on the relevant IT systems, supported by an up-to-date database of active users.

Note
Refer to Appendix 4 for supporting guidance and examples of the different subject areas individuals should be trained on in relation to their job roles, when using IT systems for the provision of equipment.

12.9 To ensure data security, all staff members appropriately trained on the use of the IT systems are issued with a secure personal identification number (PIN), or some form of approved user ID. A central database is used to hold details of 'live' users of the system, and also to keep track of changes. There is also an information sharing protocol in place and accessible to all system users. This is in keeping with organisational Data Protection and information sharing obligations.

12.10 Data cleansing policies and procedures are in use. This includes a continual update function for deceased service users.

CODE STANDARD 13

Health and Safety Management

> **OUTCOME**
> The health and safety of service users, carers, family and staff is promoted at all times, supported by clear policy, procedure and guidance.

Introduction to Code Standard 13

Health and safety is a very broad topic area, and it is most important that all relevant health and safety issues are addressed in all aspects of equipment provision, e.g. commissioning, assessment and service provision.

The potential for exposure to serious risk, e.g. electrocution, cross-contamination, is inherent with equipment services; in view of this, health and safety management should play a prominent role in the day-to-day running of equipment services.

Most of the relevant health and safety requirements relating to equipment provision are covered under the Health and Safety at Work etc. Act 1974 (HASAWA). The main aims of the HASAWA are to impose on an employer a statutory duty of care for the health, safety and welfare of its employees, and other people who may be affected by its activities, e.g. service users, the employees of contractors or members of the public.

Failure to comply with the HASAWA – whilst factoring in reasonable practicability – could result in prosecution. Serious breaches of health and safety requirements also carry the penalty of imprisonment for employees held responsible, under the Health and Safety (Offences) Act 2008.

Note that HASAWA covers all aspects of work including computer use and working conditions, etc. However, this Code of Practice is only concerned with areas specific to the provision of equipment.

Where third-party providers or suppliers are used as part of overall service provision, it is most important to ensure responsibilities are clearly defined. If they are not clear, issues may arise relating to implied terms, passage and title of risk, product liability and general product safety regulations, for example. Failure to address these issues may result in breaches of various pieces of legislation, e.g. Consumer Protection Act 1987 and the HASAWA.

Aspects of health and safety will also need to be considered when providing equipment via alternative funding options, e.g. direct payment, voucher (for wheelchairs).

13.1   There is a Health and Safety policy document covering at least the following areas:

- risk management processes – including monitoring and reviewing (Management of Health and Safety at Work Regulations 1999)
- compliance with medical device-related issues
- the Provision and Use of Work Equipment Regulations (PUWER) 1998
- the Lifting Operations and Lifting Equipment Regulations (LOLER) 1998
- the Reporting of Injuries, Diseases and Dangerous Occurrences Regulations 1995 (RIDDOR)
- competent health and safety advice.

13.2   Compliance with HASAWA requirements relating specifically to equipment can be demonstrated. Evidence of compliance with the Health and Safety Executive recommended Plan, Do, Check, Act framework, or similar approach, would be acceptable for ensuring good health and safety principles are embedded into the service.

13.3 All employees are responsible for recognising when an incident, or a near miss, has occurred, and they have a formal procedure to follow which enables them to report adverse incidents in a timely and appropriate manner.

13.4 Risk assessments are carried out as a result of any untoward incidents, and actions taken to prevent recurrence are implemented and documented on the adverse incident reports.

13.5 There is documentation clearly setting out roles and responsibilities relating to general product safety; this includes all third-party organisations responsible for providing equipment on behalf of statutory organisations.

Note
Further details relating to the HSE Plan, Do, Check, Act framework can be found here: http://www.hse.gov.uk/managing/delivering/index.htm

CODE STANDARD 14

Transportation

OUTCOME
All equipment is safely transported.

Introduction to Code Standard 14

This Code Standard relates to operational staff. The safe transportation of equipment is very important as it poses risks to the driver and to the service user. There is also the possibility of damaging the equipment while in transit. Issues arise in particular where clean and potentially contaminated equipment are transported together to and from people's homes. The Carriage of Dangerous Goods by Road Regulations 1996 place strict control on many aspects of transporting arrangements, e.g. the packaging and handling of contaminated equipment; the segregation of clean and contaminated equipment; securing of loads and safe methods of transportation.

14.1   Staff transporting equipment in their personal vehicles only do so when it is safe, without risk of cross-contamination or injury to themselves or others, and is covered formally by a suitable individual or corporate insurance policy. It may be necessary to have harnessing bolts installed in the vehicles or alternative suitable means for securing equipment, e.g. straps or a separate boot.

14.2   A policy for staff transporting equipment in personal vehicles is available, which includes a risk assessment.

14.3 Appropriate delivery mechanisms in place to ensure service users or members of the public are not unreasonably expected to collect or transport their own equipment. Exceptional circumstances may apply for small aids, but the criteria for this are clearly set out in a procedure document, and communicated to the service user, where appropriate.

14.4 Where service users are expected to collect and transport their own equipment, they are advised of and agree to the risks and are given written instructions on the best methods for transporting equipment.

14.5 There is a local policy for the management and transport of equipment from the point of use to the decontamination facility; this may be part of a wider organisational transport policy.

14.6 Vehicles used for transporting contaminated equipment are made of suitable material which allows the vehicle to be satisfactorily cleaned.

14.7 Vehicles used for transporting both clean and contaminated equipment have appropriate segregation controls in use, which also comply with local infection control policy.

14.8 Vehicles used for transporting equipment are of an appropriate size and shape to accommodate the various equipment types, e.g. beds, hoists and wheelchairs, and have appropriate adaptations, e.g. ramps, lifts, where appropriate, to safely transport equipment.

14.9 Vehicles used for transporting equipment are suitably equipped with gloves, aprons, bags for contaminated equipment, and cleaning agents for hands, etc.

14.10 Appropriate hazard warning signs are displayed on vehicles, e.g. heavy loads, contaminated equipment, hazardous materials.

14.11 Vehicles used for transporting equipment are maintained regularly to ensure that they are safe and fit for purpose, with appropriate records kept.

CODE STANDARD 15

Decontamination

> **OUTCOME**
> Service users and staff are kept safe and free from contamination or infection by ensuring decontamination of all equipment, medical devices, facilities and vehicles is properly managed.

Introduction to Code Standard 15

Where equipment is loaned to service users and brought back in for reuse when no longer required, the potential for cross-infection is one of the greatest service user safety concerns. Compliance with MHRA Medical Device guidance on decontamination should be followed to ensure risks of contamination and cross-infection are minimised. It is very important to ensure all equipment is decontaminated before being reissued to another service user.

15.1   To ensure the safety of service users, carers and staff, there are appropriate systems in place so that all reusable equipment and medical devices are properly decontaminated prior to use or repair, and that the risks associated with decontamination facilities and processes are well managed.

15.2   The assumption is made that all reused equipment and medical devices are contaminated, and staff take precautions to reduce the risk to themselves and others, e.g. use of safe systems of work, personal and suitable protective equipment and/or clothing.

15.3 All equipment and medical devices are decontaminated and stored in accordance with legislative and best practice requirements, e.g. manufacturer's guidance, MHRA guidance.

15.4 Dedicated and suitable facilities are used for decontaminating equipment. These facilities are of a suitable size in proportion to the activity requirements and throughput. They are easily accessible, with complete segregation from clean equipment.

15.5 Local protocols are in place to consider decontamination requirements before reusable equipment and medical devices are acquired, to ensure they are compatible with the decontamination equipment available. Examples of those to be included in the protocol for consultation, or for generally seeking advice, include:

- manufacturer of device
- manufacturer of decontamination/reprocessing equipment
- infection control staff
- consultant microbiologist or consultant in communicable disease
- competent health and safety advisers
- device and equipment users
- advice from MHRA
- in-house technical/decontamination staff
- clinical professionals.

15.6 There are different methods of decontamination used to address varying levels of contamination, depending on the equipment/device, risk assessment classification and its use. The methods of decontamination could include: cleaning, cleaning followed by disinfection and/or sterilization. A protocol is in place which describes the type of equipment and suitable decontamination processes.

Note
Refer to supporting guidance in Appendix 6 relating to classification of

infection risk together with the recommendations for appropriate decontamination treatments.

15.7 Where third-party contractors carry out cleaning and decontamination functions on behalf of equipment providers, a detailed service specification covering all aspects of decontamination is in place. Equipment returned from third-party contractors is labelled with a certificate, or clearly marked, to demonstrate it has been appropriately decontaminated.

15.8 Regardless of where equipment has been in the system, e.g. subject to inspection, maintenance, or repair, either on site or at the manufacturer's premises, it is decontaminated before being returned to stock available for issue. Equipment is decontaminated prior to being scrapped.

15.9 Any loaned equipment, or equipment on trial being returned to a manufacturer or supplier, is decontaminated with appropriate certification attached.

15.10 When equipment has been appropriately decontaminated it is labelled, or clearly marked, accordingly and, where appropriate, a declaration of contamination status form is completed. This is readily accessible to the recipient of the equipment. Electronic tracking information also highlights the decontamination status of each piece of equipment.

15.11 Chemicals used are compatible with the device and at the correct concentration as recommended by the various manufacturers involved.

15.12 The decontamination equipment used to clean equipment is properly commissioned and validated. It is also subject to planned maintenance by properly trained and competent staff. Maintenance records are available for assessment.

15.13 Staff expected to carry out decontamination are:

- appropriately trained
- aware of needle sticks and sharps injury procedures
- provided with suitable equipment/clothing
- made aware of legal requirements
- able to access policies and procedures.

15.14 Should the user or carer be expected to decontaminate equipment, before disposal for example, appropriate information and equipment, e.g. bags and gloves, are provided.

15.15 There is a senior member of staff and single point of contact to manage and communicate all aspects of decontamination. The decontamination procedures are clearly understood at all levels throughout the provider organisation.

15.16 There are clear lines of responsibility for decontamination matters across the organisation, leading to the relevant management board or group.

15.17 Senior managers and/or the relevant management board/group monitor and regularly review decontamination procedures through audit. This is documented and sent to the appropriate management board/group, and/or appropriate health and safety, or risk, officer for sign-off.

CODE STANDARD 16

Performance Management

OUTCOME
Performance is linked to and can be measured against individual
and organisational aims and objectives.

Introduction to Code Standard 16

Performance management includes activities which ensure that aims and
objectives are consistently being met in an effective and efficient manner.
Performance management not only focuses on the performance of an
organisation, but on departments, services and employees, as well as other
areas.

As with any service or contract, it is most important to ensure relevant
performance measures are in place to capture the overall performance of
service provision. Performance standards will generally be set by those with
commissioning responsibilities, although these will also have to be agreed
by the provider to ensure they are realistic and achievable, and that they can
be measured effectively.

Providers will also have their own performance-related standards and
objectives so that they can manage internal performance, especially where
there is dependence upon third-party contractors to deliver.

For some years, equipment providers have produced reports on a variety of statistical type key performance indicators (KPIs). Whilst these reports are useful, they can be considered 'one dimensional' and do not necessarily portray the whole picture. Performance needs to be contextualized. It is important that any key performance indicator-style reporting is backed up with, and complemented by, reporting on the overall outcomes of the service. This helps to put any KPIs in context.

16.1   There are robust reporting mechanisms in place in order to satisfy commissioners and internal and external auditors that performance, including that of third-party providers or suppliers, can be assessed and is at an acceptable level.

16.2   Various performance reports are available which cover key areas of the service. Examples of these include, but are not limited to:

- key performance indicators (KPIs) management reports, e.g. time taken from referral to prescription to delivery of equipment
- response times to client, urgent and standard
- reasons for failing to deliver equipment within agreed timescale
- waiting lists, or unredeemed prescriptions or vouchers
- stock value, turnaround, write-offs, collection rates and recycling levels
- number of assets requiring maintenance. This may include urgent repair targets
- third-party supplier performance, e.g. lead times
- savings achieved
- cost saving strategies through improved recall systems, recycling and improved maintenance schedule
- health and safety action plan
- findings from risk assessments
- number of accolades and complaints
- number of near misses/incidents/investigations
- service user satisfaction surveys
- staff turnover levels
- infection control (random spot checks)
- quality control processes in place, e.g. policies and procedures.

16.3   If performance falls below an acceptable standard, this can be identified in a timely way and can be proactively managed to ensure performance levels are restored.

16.4   Managing performance is seen as a continuous process which involves making sure that the performance of employees contributes to the aims and objectives of the service. This may be, for example, letting employees know what the service is trying to achieve, their role in helping the service achieve its goals and providing them with the skill and competencies they need to fulfil their role.

16.5   Employees have regular performance reviews and these consider the standards of performance required from them, how they can develop their individual performance and contribute to the development of the service, and how they are performing.

CODE STANDARD 17

Emergency and Out-of-hours Cover

> **OUTCOME**
> Service users or their carers will at all times have access to emergency repairs or replacement of equipment, where appropriate.

Introduction to Code Standard 17

Some equipment is highly technical and requires regular maintenance. Occasionally equipment needs to be repaired, or in some cases replaced. It is important that service users are able to obtain a repair or replacement for certain types of equipment at any time, even out of hours or on a public holiday, particularly if the service user or their carer is completely dependent upon the equipment, e.g. hoist or wheelchair, as without it their or their carer's health and wellbeing could be at risk.

It is obviously not viable for providers to be available at any time of the day or night, seven days a week, all year. It is, however, possible to ensure that service users have at least a contact number where concerns can be discussed and dealt with as appropriate.

17.1 Appropriate risk assessments are undertaken to identify which pieces of equipment have emergency cover available out of hours. These assessments factor in such things as the service user's vulnerability, independence and mobility, for example.

17.2   For equipment identified under clause 17.1, there is emergency cover in place at all times for service users in the event of equipment breakdown, to include: normal working hours; outside normal working hours; weekends, and public holidays.

17.3   Where appropriate, cover is in the form of repair (either in the service user's home or at the provider's premises), or replacement of the equipment, where practicable. Where repair or replacement is not an immediate option, procedures are in place to ensure the service user and/or their carer is made safe until the equipment can be repaired properly or replaced.

17.4   All service users are provided with contact details and instructions should problems arise with their equipment; this includes an out-of-hours telephone helpline number, and a troubleshooting checklist for their equipment, if appropriate.

17.5   Consideration is given to how service users that receive their equipment via an alternative funding option, e.g. direct payment or voucher, might be supported in the event of an equipment breakdown. This will depend on the conditions originally agreed to when the funding for equipment was awarded.

CODE STANDARD 18

Stock Management

> **OUTCOME**
> Stock is managed efficiently whilst ensuring optimum output is achieved at all times.

Introduction to Code Standard 18

Having appropriate levels of stock in place, and being able to source equipment in a timely manner, is crucial for effective equipment provision, especially where being out of stock, or not able to source equipment, could result in, for example, someone being admitted to hospital.

It is important for services to ensure that arrangements are in place to include back-up systems detailing alternative products in the event that certain product lines are not in stock, or cannot be obtained easily. Holding adequate stock does, however, have to be balanced with acquisition and stock holding costs.

Whilst stock management is generally considered to only be relevant to products that are 'stock' items, it is also important that robust procurement arrangements are in place for some of the more 'complex' and 'non-routine' items.

18.1   There is a robust (ideally electronic) stock control system in place, with a designated lead responsible for managing stock levels.

18.2   Appropriate safety stock levels are in place within stores for ensuring the likelihood of running out of stock is minimised, with suitable back-up systems in place providing alternative (clinically approved) products, where certain product lines are not in stock.

18.3   There are robust arrangements in place to ensure 'complex' and 'non-routine' items and parts, can be obtained in a timely manner.

18.4   Regular cyclical stock audits are in place with reconciliation updates on the stock management system, where necessary. The procedure for dealing with shortfalls is written into an appropriate 'Writing Off' or 'Disposal' policy.

18.5   Where third-party providers or suppliers are used as part of core provision, steps are taken to ensure stock management issues, including lead times and stock levels, are formally addressed.

CODE STANDARD 19

Recycling

OUTCOME
Equipment lifespan and levels of recycling are maximised through efficient collection procedures, appropriate servicing, maintenance, decontamination and refurbishing of equipment.

Introduction to Code Standard 19

Recycling is a fundamental and efficient part of the overall provision of equipment. As equipment is issued on loan, inevitably equipment will come back into the service for reuse. An efficient service will maximise recycling levels in preference to purchasing new equipment as this can represent a significant cost saving, and ensures more people can receive equipment. This is particularly important for complex and specialist equipment, which is not only generally difficult to acquire, but is also usually very expensive. However, equipment should never be reissued once it has been in use for its recommended useful life, as per the manufacturer's guidance, as this poses serious risks for service users.

19.1   All returned equipment is cleaned and refurbished to a standard which meets manufacturers', health and safety, Medicines and Healthcare Products Regulatory Agency (MHRA), and infection control requirements, before being reissued. Consideration is also given to the method of suitable repackaging, where appropriate.

Note

MHRA have developed all the necessary information required for decontaminating equipment: MHRA (2006). Managing Medical Devices. *Guidance for healthcare and social services organisations.* DB2006 (05) only available on website: www.mhra.gov.uk. MHRA (2003). *Community Equipment Loan Stores – Guidance on Decontamination*, DB2003 (06).

19.2   Equipment is only recycled for reuse if it is within its manufacturer's recommended lifespan. Any equipment which has been in use for longer than its recommended lifespan is written off.

19.3   A recycling policy is in place for ensuring a quality, cost-effective service for the servicing, maintenance, decontamination and refurbishing of equipment in order that the equipment lifespan is optimised, accounting for both the number of cycles of use and maximum number of years in use. The policy should cover, but should not necessarily be limited to:

- recycling instructions
- recycling performance levels
- collection performance levels
- scrapping and 'writing off' policy
- salvaging equipment for parts
- guidance on repair, refurbishment and modifications.

Note

'Recycling' incorporates the retrieval, cleaning and decontamination, maintenance, repair and refurbishment, so that equipment is fit for reissue.

CODE STANDARD 20

Assembling, Fitting and Demonstrating Equipment

> **OUTCOME**
> Equipment is safely assembled, fitted and demonstrated by competent staff.

Introduction to Code Standard 20

There is a vast range of equipment, with differing levels of complexity in terms of assembly, fitting and demonstration requirements. For example, while there is not a great deal of technical input required when issuing a walking frame, a profiling bed with a high-risk pressure mattress, or a complex wheelchair, requires very careful assembly, fitting or adjustment, and demonstration.

Equipment poorly assembled and fitted can be very dangerous, and there are cases where this has resulted in serious incidents and fatalities. This aspect of service delivery should be given due care and attention, when considering roles, responsibilities, competencies and training requirements.

This section is also directly relevant where third-party providers or suppliers are used, as some of these are expected to assemble, fit and demonstrate equipment.

20.1 All staff delivering equipment which requires assembling and fitting are suitably trained and qualified to do so.

20.2   Training and information provided to service users, and/or their carers or family, is appropriate to the complexity of the equipment to be assembled, fitted and demonstrated, and it considers the individual needs of the person using the equipment, including their abilities to use the equipment, together with the environment in which the equipment is to be used.

20.3   Written procedures are in place outlining the correct processes to be followed for installation, fitting and demonstrating equipment. These include, but are not limited to:

- equipment types, and the different levels of training and qualifications required
- use of manufacturers' and/or in-house written instructions for users
- warnings and safety notices
- building structure and load-bearing considerations
- access to and from the environment/s where the equipment is to be used
- demonstration for the service user and/or carer, including: verbal explanations, the correct use of the equipment in-situ, responding to any questions, queries, or concerns raised by the service user.

20.4   Equipment is installed, fitted and/or adjusted, in accordance with the manufacturer's instructions, and complies with specifications supplied by the original clinical prescriber.

20.5   Where necessary, staff have the appropriate communication skills and training to enable them to advise service users and carers on safe use of equipment. This training should include communication tactics with deaf and hard of hearing people, and people with vision impairments.

20.6   Where appropriate, service users, carers and families are part of any dialogue and decisions relating to the installation, fitting and/or adjusting of the equipment. This may form part of a risk assessment which outlines the capacity of the individual or carer to understand the training/demonstration and the potential need to offer written advice and training. This is especially important for children, and those with limited abilities, when using complex equipment, especially where high risk is present, e.g. a powered wheelchair. Notification that a demonstration of the equipment has been received is documented and, where appropriate, put on the service user's patient record.

20.7   At each delivery, staff unpack the equipment, safely removing all wrapping and packaging, and leave any specific manufacturers', or otherwise approved, instructions for clinicians, technicians, carers, or service users, as appropriate.

CODE STANDARD 21

Minor Adaptations

> **OUTCOME**
> Adaptations are accessible and safely carried out by competent staff.

Introduction to Code Standard 21

Minor adaptations generally refer to minor alterations made to a service user's property. Adaptations are for the purpose of increasing or maintaining functional independence to enable the service user to access and remain in their own home, to ensure safety and/or to assist carers by minimising the physical demands placed on them.

Some of the areas where adaptations may be necessary include, but are not limited to:

- household and environmental fittings, e.g. curtain and window openers
- access, e.g. grab rails, portable ramps, door fitments.

Equipment providers will usually have, or work in conjunction with, technicians. These technicians will be trained in the process for carrying out minor adaptations, and similar duties.

Some third-party providers and suppliers install simple aids to daily living, e.g. grab rails, toilet surrounds. It is very important, therefore, that where these duties are undertaken on behalf of statutory bodies, by third parties, a risk assessment has been undertaken and that the third parties have been provided with, or are required to already have, the appropriate skills and training necessary for undertaking the task.

21.1 There is clear guidance in place, including eligibility criteria, about a service user's entitlement to home adaptations.

21.2 Provision of adaptations only takes place following an individual assessment of need by an occupational therapist, occupational therapy assistant or other suitably qualified therapist, assessor or technician.

21.3 There are formal checks in place to ensure those undertaking home adaptations are suitably qualified to do so; this applies to internal and external (third-party) providers.

21.4 Where an adaptation is required, a process seeking formal agreement is followed. This may include the service user, carer, other members of the household, and other appropriate agencies.

21.5 Where appropriate, service users, carers and families are part of any dialogue and decisions relating to the installation, fitting and/or adjusting of the equipment.

21.6 Where adaptations are required urgently, there is a process in place to ensure these can be fast-tracked.

21.7 Following the installation of a minor adaptation, appropriate quality checks are made to ensure all fitness for purpose, quality and safety requirements have been fully met. Checks are carried out by someone competent to do so.

CODE STANDARD 22

Manual Handling

> **OUTCOME**
> Manual handling processes are in place to ensure risks are minimised and safety is a priority for staff, carers and service users.

Introduction to Code Standard 22

The provision of equipment often involves a series of manual handling tasks. For example, equipment will need to be manually handled within a store, or when staff deliver, install, or maintain equipment. This may also involve heavy equipment being manually handled upstairs in service users' homes, e.g. beds, hoists. Equipment is also regularly manually handled by service users and carers.

As Manual Handling Operations Regulations 1992 apply to all stakeholders and providers of the service, individual partners, service providers (including third-party contractors), and employees (including clinical professionals), all are responsible for ensuring manual handling risks are minimised and, where possible, avoided, which could otherwise result in injury.

22.1 Safe handling procedures are in place to ensure manual handling risks are minimised and safety is a priority for staff and service users.

22.2   Staff are trained and kept up to date on relevant manual handling procedures. Where manual handling cannot be avoided, a suitable and sufficient risk assessment is carried out, including the task, load, working environment, physical capabilities of the staff, service users and carers involved, and any other relevant factors.

22.3   Where equipment is provided to reduce the risks involved in manual handling, e.g. hoists, slings, and electric profiling beds, adequate training, information and instructions on the use of the equipment are provided to the service user or carer; this is documented and signed as complete by the service user or their representative.

CODE STANDARD 23

Medical Device Management

> **OUTCOME**
> Equipment is safe and effective, and risks to service users and others through use of equipment are minimised.

Introduction to Code Standard 23

The purpose of good medical device management is to ensure equipment is safe and effective. This is achieved by having a systematic and comprehensive approach to the acquisition, deployment, maintenance (including preventive maintenance), repair and disposal of medical devices, and medical device training.

Good medical device management is a fundamental part of providing safe and good quality care. Failure to ensure medical devices are managed appropriately has resulted in many adverse incidents and even fatalities over recent years. It is essential that medical device management procedures are available and followed as a matter of course, wherever equipment is provided.

23.1 There is policy documentation, and operating procedures, specifically relating to medical device management, covering the following subjects:

- policies and procedures

- reporting incidents
- Medical Device Management Board/Group, e.g. responsibilities
- acquisition processes
- electrical safety testing
- repair and maintenance
- training for clinical and technical staff and service users
- information and record management, e.g. user instructions
- decontamination and disposal processes.

Third-party providers and suppliers should also be working to similar medical device operating procedures.

Note
Refer to Supporting Criteria in Appendix 5 when considering the above headings.

23.2   There are clear lines of accountability throughout the provider organisation, supported by procedures, leading to the relevant commissioning group, including the process for managing medical device alerts.

23.3   There is a designated individual with ultimate responsibility for ensuring what is requested by the Medical Device Management Board/Group or relevant commissioning authority, is being delivered. This individual is also responsible for highlighting to the relevant group or authority any problems that arise with equipment.

23.4   There are performance and quality reports available to support medical device management, with a particular emphasis upon planned preventative maintenance.

PART THREE

CLINICAL AND PROFESSIONAL RESPONSIBILITIES

Introduction to Code Standards 24 to 35

This part mainly addresses the standards clinical professionals should be working to when assessing for and prescribing equipment. It is recognised that some technical staff will be part of the assessment process, and this Part applies equally to them.

Some organisations occasionally require third-party providers and suppliers to undertake certain assessment and prescribing tasks on their behalf, and these activities are also covered in this Part.

This section is not intended to replace, recreate or conflict with any professional standards clinical or technical practitioners are currently working to as part of their professional code of conduct.

Where clinical activities are an intrinsic part of stores operations, as in some wheelchair and seating services, for example, then this Part is to be read in conjunction with Part 2, Service Provision.

When professionals assess for and prescribe equipment they are expected to adhere to various governing standards and regulations. For example, besides having to meet the standards of their respective councils and professional bodies, they are required to work within organisational and regulatory boundaries. They are also expected to work in coordination with the providers of equipment services. With these issues in mind this Part carefully pulls together the various obligations of professionals, with regard to equipment.

For there to be a safe and effective service provided to the service user, collaboration is required between those undertaking the assessments and the equipment provider.

CODE STANDARD 24

Assessing the Service User's Equipment Needs

> **OUTCOME**
> There is a clear, comprehensive, easy to follow, and consistent service user assessment procedure in place which enables all service users' equipment needs to be identified satisfactorily.

Introduction to Code Standard 24

This standard considers the various aspects associated with the service user assessment process, with regards to the provision of equipment.

The assessment process is generally straightforward when there is the requirement for a single basic piece of equipment, and where there is only one assessment to meet a particular need. Complications can ensue, however, when, for example, a service user has multiple needs, and especially where some of their requirements are for complex equipment, e.g. major adaptations to the home, or complex wheelchair, posture and seating requirements. These difficulties can be compounded where, for example, several clinicians carry out different assessments to meet different health, social care and education-related needs.

Assessments should also look beyond the immediate need of the service user and consider wider implications of their health condition, such as the risk of developing body shape distortions through remaining too long in one position, for example.

Regardless of the service users' needs, it is important to ensure there is an all-embracing, holistic and consistent process applied when assessing the service user, to ensure the full range of their needs are sufficiently met, and that staff are competent to carry out the assessments.

It is also important that the views of the service user are sought and form part of the assessment as a matter of course.

24.1 There is a clear referral pathway into the service. Referrals are triaged and managed appropriately and in a timely manner, taking into account priority of need, with clear decision making and communication processes, either to offer advice and support, signpost to other provision or accept the referral for assessment.

24.2 There is a simple and structured (preferably electronic) process in place to receive and collate referral information. This should link to a database of existing service users, so that it is possible to check information already held about the service user, and whether other clinical professionals are involved in the case.

24.3 Appropriate screening processes are in place, reflecting appropriate levels of seniority for various levels of need. Screening also includes:

- a process for collecting additional information, where necessary, and ensuring any gaps in the referral data are appropriately dealt with and updated
- a process for dealing with paper and face-to-face assessments
- a process for allocating assessors, including urgent need, particularly for those with rapidly progressing conditions and terminal illnesses.

24.4 Once the equipment needs have been assessed, outcomes, options and decisions are discussed with appropriate authorities, and with the service user or carer, and appropriately documented and communicated; this also reflects the necessary levels of authorisation.

24.5 A policy document or procedure clearly sets out the process for assessment and provision of:

- standard and routine equipment (including involvement of third-party providers, where appropriate)
- non-standard equipment, e.g. beds and hoists
- complex and specialist equipment, e.g. bariatric and children's equipment, including wheelchairs and seating
- minor adaptations
- major adaptations.

24.6 Any assessment of equipment needs is person-centred, anticipatory and conducted in the context of a multidisciplinary or integrated team, where appropriate.

24.7 Assessments for equipment factor in the whole-life, and changing, needs of the service user, including anticipatory and reasonable lifestyle needs, and not just the clinical need, e.g. can the user or carer use the equipment now and in the future; can the equipment be used outside, and is it safe in situ.

24.8 Assessments consider those associated with the service user, such as family, carers, guardians, teachers, allied healthcare professionals, etc., and the environment in which the service user lives and often frequents (including the home, education, work and leisure).

24.9 Any unmet equipment needs and/or any unresolved issues or disagreements are recorded, as part of the assessment.

24.10 All assessments, including specialist and complex, for children and adults, are conducted in accordance with evidence-based national or local good practice guidelines, where these exist.

24.11 Service users are offered assessments either by telephone and/or letter, and are seen either in a clinical, home, school, or work environment dependant on the service user's specified needs.

24.12 Any training needs for the service user and/or their carer are identified as part of the assessment process.

24.13 There is a process in place to allow the original assessor to know that the equipment provision is completed; this includes third-party provision, and where equipment is provided via an alternative funding route, e.g. personal budget or voucher (for wheelchairs), as appropriate. This prompts arrangements for a review to be carried out to check that the equipment meets the needs.

24.14 Depending on the service user's situation and the type of equipment/adaptations provided, the assessor sets a review date based on clinical risk assessment, to ensure the equipment is still meeting the service user's needs, e.g. after one year. As a result, this could lead to more assessment, more services, removal or replacement of equipment, or closure of the case.

CODE STANDARD 25

Managing Multiple Assessments

> **OUTCOME**
> Multiple assessments are coordinated and, where possible, reduced to avoid duplication and delays, and to minimise the number of contacts for service users.

Introduction to Code Standard 25

Many service users require a range of equipment, and as a result they receive multiple assessments, often from different clinical teams, disciplines, and services, in order to meet all of their needs. This can be frustrating for the service user, especially those with rapidly progressing conditions and terminal illnesses, as they will have many contacts with different services, and there are inevitably delays.

If multiple assessments are not managed properly and, where appropriate, reduced, this results in duplication, inefficiency, delays and various pieces of equipment arriving at different times.

To address these issues, the processes around multiple assessments should be coordinated in a systematic and timely manner and, where possible, the number of contacts reduced; ideally this should be through a single-assessment, or similar process.

With some service users now having access to and a need for a wide range of equipment services and advancing technologies, there needs to be a shift in thinking about how people are assessed. For example, staff could be trained in undertaking more 'holistic' assistive technology-related assessments. Obviously there would sometimes still need to be specialist assessments for complex cases.

Some traditional assessment models may actually be going against the direction of person-centred care, where the service user has to try to fit in with the different service models; this can result in poor outcomes and experiences for service users and their carers.

Whilst reducing the number of contacts for the service user, and closer working, requires the efforts of different teams and services, it is essential for this firstly to be supported by formal agreements between the relevant commissioning authorities to allow this to happen.

25.1 A policy or process is in place to demonstrate that service users receive safe, seamless, timely and coordinated assessments, care, treatment and support when more than one provider or specialist is involved, or when they move between services.

25.2 A multi-agency protocol exists to reflect the approach to be taken where different pieces of equipment are necessary to meet a range of needs. This includes any dialogue and communication requirements with the service user and/or carer, and, where appropriate, third-party (partner) organisations.

25.3 Services are prioritised for people with urgent equipment needs, e.g. those with rapidly progressing conditions or terminal illnesses, to ensure equipment is made available quickly and the number of assessments and contacts with the service user are kept to a minimum.

25.4 Efforts are made to provide more 'holistic' assessments, so that a wide range of equipment-related needs can be assessed for and met in the most efficient and timely manner.

25.5   Services provided by all relevant parties are coordinated and work together in a timely manner, making efforts to ensure the service user has a minimal number of contacts.

25.6   Information about the service user can be accessed and shared easily across different services and agencies; this respects data protection issues.

CODE STANDARD 26

Assessing the Home and Environment

> **OUTCOME**
> Assessments of the home and environment are carried out thoroughly, in a timely and consistent manner.

Introduction to Code Standard 26

Equipment can be required for use in a single setting, or it may be required for use in a range of settings, e.g. home, education, work and leisure.

When assessing a service user for the equipment they need, it is essential to take into account where they will need to use this equipment; in many cases an assessment of the home will be necessary to ensure suitability of the equipment.

Problems can arise if staff assessing a service user fail to take into account such things as: other furniture already in the house; specific dimensions and accessibility of the house or room, e.g. steps, stairs or ramps. It can also be problematic when hospital-based staff discharge service users with equipment into the community, without having physically assessed the home or their environment.

It is important also for an assessment to consider settings other than the home, where the equipment is likely to be used. This is particularly important for people using wheelchairs.

26.1 Where assessments of the home and/or the environment where the equipment is to be used are undertaken, this includes a standardised risk assessment which enables all reasonable eventualities of risk or harm to be identified, minimised, or removed. A dialogue will also be necessary, in some instances, with the service user and/or carer.

26.2 There is guidance, e.g. local discharge policy, setting out the process to be followed where a physical assessment of the home or environment is required; this guidance also specifies which equipment types require an assessment.

26.3 Assessments of the home and the settings where equipment is to be used consider the whole-life needs of the service user and not just the clinical needs, e.g. Can the equipment be used in certain rooms? Can the equipment be used outdoors? How does the equipment impact upon other members of the family? Assessments of the home or environment also have input from the service user and/or carer, or family members, as a matter of course.

26.4 Where the same piece of equipment is required in different settings, consideration is given to this when undertaking the assessment of the home or environment, including, for example, how the equipment will be transported.

26.5 Where third-party providers are used, they have been provided with clear instructions relating to findings from home and environmental assessments, including, where appropriate, issues which may impact upon delivery and fitting arrangements.

CODE STANDARD 27

Training in Equipment Provision and Use

> **OUTCOME**
> Appropriate training is undertaken with regards to provision and use of equipment, and this is carried out by competent individuals and is supplemented by written information.

Introduction to Code Standard 27

This particular Code Standard relates generally to clinical professionals, but certain aspects may be relevant to some technical staff.

Training on the various aspects of equipment provision and use, is an area that can easily be overlooked. It is sometimes assumed that because someone has a clinical, or technical, background they do not need any training on equipment.

It is critical for staff to understand the technical functions of equipment and how these meet the clinical needs of the service user. This is especially important where complex or even life-supporting equipment is provided.

Where third-party providers and suppliers are used to undertake certain tasks on behalf of organisations, training requirements will also need to be considered.

The Medicines and Healthcare Products Regulatory Agency (MHRA) has emphasized the importance of appropriate training in its guidance *Managing Medical Devices*, and has detailed the considerations to be given for each role. It has stated that all aspects of training in relation to service provision should be incorporated into a policy document which should be developed by the medical devices management group, should one exist; see Appendix 5 for further details.

27.1 A policy document exists which specifies responsibilities for training, together with procedures to be followed for training on equipment provided, both to clinical professionals, technicians, third-party providers and suppliers, and to service users and/or carers (where appropriate).

27.2 Those responsible for prescribing equipment are given relevant training by competent individuals, to ensure that they understand how the manufacturer intends the product to be used and that they can relay to the service user and/or carer the intended use and functions of the device in order to use it safely, and maximise its performance.

27.3 Those with responsibilities for providing equipment ensure that they are appropriately trained and kept up to date on the specific equipment categories they issue. For example, this may be achieved through a Continuing Professional Development programme.

27.4 Clinical and professional staff work to suitable and recognised competencies, and these reflect their seniority and the complexity of the equipment they provide.

27.5 Appropriate training and support information, e.g. manufacturers' instructions, are made available and communicated to staff and service users, as appropriate.

27.6 A structure is in place demonstrating the different levels of equipment that can be ordered and provided by the different grades of staff; this will usually be based upon complexity of equipment, and in some cases financial thresholds.

27.7 Where necessary, staff, including third-party providers and suppliers, have the appropriate communication skills and training to enable them to advise service users or carers on safe use of equipment. This training should include communication tactics with deaf and hard of hearing people, and people with visual impairments.

Note
With regards to wheelchair and seating services, information about training and relevant courses can be found on the Posture and Mobility Group website: www.pmguk.co.uk.

CODE STANDARD 28

Transportation of Equipment

> **OUTCOME**
> All equipment is safely transported, with minimal risk to clinicians, service users, carers and others.

Introduction to Code Standard 28

This Code Standard relates mainly to clinical staff. Clinical staff should not be expected to regularly deliver and collect equipment in their personal vehicles. Some organisations provide vehicles for transporting equipment; it is recognised, however, that in some instances clinical staff may need to transport equipment. Where equipment is transported in personal vehicles, this presents some risks which should be given careful consideration. The following list sets out some examples of the risks to be considered:

- transportation of clean and contaminated equipment in the same vehicle carries the risk of cross-contamination, and consequently infecting service users
- clinical staff may not be fully insured to carry equipment in their personal vehicles
- clinical staff could expose themselves to personal injury.

In some instances third-party providers and suppliers are asked to deliver equipment to service users. Where this is the case, it is important that due regard is given to safe transportation issues.

28.1 Clinical staff are never required to carry contaminated equipment in their personal vehicles. This includes equipment used for assessment purposes.

28.2 Where clinical staff deliver clean equipment in their personal vehicles, this is only done where:

- necessary adjustments have been made to vehicles, e.g. secure fixing points
- individuals are properly insured
- a formal risk assessment has been undertaken.

28.3 All of the above issues are reflected in a policy document. This may form part of a larger transport policy.

CODE STANDARD 29

Selecting and Purchasing Equipment

> **OUTCOME**
> There are clear clinical criteria and a consistent process used for selecting and acquiring equipment, which take into consideration both the organisation's and the service user's needs.

Introduction to Code Standard 29

Although most equipment acquisitions are made by the equipment provider or store, clinical staff and teams are usually involved in selection of equipment, and sometimes have purchasing responsibilities for certain types of equipment. This Code Standard relates to the role of clinical staff, whether procuring equipment themselves, or working with providers in the selection process. It follows that the evidence to support this Code Standard may be found with the clinical teams and/or with the equipment service (store).

It is vital that service users receive the right equipment which is best suited to meet their needs. For this reason it is essential for clinical staff to be involved in the selection of equipment for purchase, as they have a better understanding of each service user's needs, and the products available on the market to meet these needs. It does not necessarily follow that the 'best' (and often most expensive) product in the market is the most suitable piece of equipment for the service user.

There should be a formal procurement process to go through when selecting new equipment, to ensure all safety, quality and suitability issues are addressed. The process should align with local organisational policies, e.g. best value. The process could be defined within the terms of reference of a product selection group, for example.

The equipment selection process should have appropriate representation, e.g. store managers, technicians, service users, clinical, and procurement professionals, to ensure all views are considered and processes adhered to. There should be sufficient expertise available to provide ongoing support and maintenance for any equipment acquired.

Where national procurement frameworks and catalogues are available to choose equipment from, these will generally have already been through a robust equipment selection process, using appropriate criteria. However, before using equipment from the agreed national frameworks and catalogues it is important for local areas to ensure that they are satisfied with the equipment selection process which has been used, as this may not comply with internal governance and medical device management policies and procedures.

29.1 All equipment selections are based primarily upon formal clinical criteria, i.e. where the service user's needs are paramount, whilst also taking into account other relevant factors.

29.2 A policy or procedure is in place to ensure the selection and purchase of new equipment addresses safety, quality, and performance issues, and that it represents best value. This also includes equipment acquired from any national frameworks or catalogues.

29.3 Policies and procedures for selecting and purchasing new equipment include and take account of the needs and preferences of all interested parties, e.g. stores, commissioning, procurement, decontamination, maintenance, the service user, carer and prescribing clinicians.

29.4 Policies and procedures for purchasing equipment align with and support any approved local or national contracts, or frameworks, in place, as these will usually have undergone a rigorous supplier and product vetting and evaluation process.

29.5　All new acquisitions are made through appropriate procurement channels, e.g. non-standard processes and products are approved by a product selection group.

29.6　The staff responsible for selecting and purchasing new equipment have appropriate links with the medical device, or suitable equipment, board/group, where one exists.

29.7　There is a procedure in place for any instances where staff operate outside the normal equipment selection process, e.g. when only one product is on the market to meet a specific need.

29.8　Issues such as supplier lead times, availability and costs of replacement parts, the decontamination requirements and recyclability of equipment, are considered before equipment is purchased.

29.9　Consideration is given to how service users and their carers might be supported, e.g. signposting services, or in acquiring equipment when it is offered or chosen outside the normal channels of provision, e.g. direct payment, personal budgets or vouchers (for wheelchairs).

CODE STANDARD 30

Demonstrating and Trialling Complex, Specialist and Children's Equipment

> **OUTCOME**
> Equipment is demonstrated and trialled appropriately and in a safe and suitable environment.

Introduction to Code Standard 30

The opportunity to try out a piece of equipment is important to a lot of service users, and is helpful as part of the process for ensuring it meets the user's needs. It is also an obvious area where user involvement is appropriate.

Demonstrating equipment appropriately can sometimes pose problems, particularly if there are inappropriate facilities, or if the user has mobility problems. Often, staff physically take equipment to service users' homes, or schools; alternatively service users have to visit an equipment store or a dedicated demonstration facility.

Some equipment suppliers also provide demonstrations of equipment at service users' homes, particularly for children's equipment. Although this approach has some advantages, particularly for individuals who feel most comfortable in familiar surroundings, there can be unnecessary delays, particularly if the equipment is not suitable and the service user needs alternative equipment demonstrated, for example.

Sometimes equipment can be left with the service user for trialling, as longer periods can be required with certain products to assess suitability, etc. This, however, is not without problems, e.g. breakdown cover and maintenance responsibilities. Issues relating to obligations and accountability need to be clear, in the event of something going wrong when the equipment is on trial with the service user.

It is important for trials and demonstrations of equipment to take place in the right environment, and in the place where the service user feels most comfortable, and is most likely to be using the equipment on a regular basis, e.g. home or school.

30.1   There are appropriate facilities available for service users, carers, and staff to have equipment suitably and safely demonstrated. There is a policy or procedure in place supporting this, stating what equipment is available for trial and the various locations this can take place, e.g. an equipment store, demonstration centre, home, school.

30.2   Where service users are not able to access the demonstration facilities, a suitable appointment is arranged to allow equipment to be appropriately demonstrated and/or trialled.

30.3   Where equipment is on loan or trial for assessment purposes, including from a supplier, it is made clear whose responsibility it will be should any problems arise.

30.4   Risk assessments are undertaken where trials and demonstrations take place, to reduce the likelihood of an incident occurring.

CODE STANDARD 31

Equipment-related Risk Assessments

> **OUTCOME**
> Risks and potential hazards relating to equipment are identified, prevented or reduced, documented, communicated and managed in a timely and systematic manner.

Introduction to Code Standard 31

In an equipment service, responsibility for assessing and managing risk is shared between commissioners and providers, including clinical and technical staff. This Code Standard is principally taken up with responsibilities of clinical staff, although some aspects do touch on the responsibilities of technical staff and third-party providers.

It is important to note that although there are separate clinical, technical and provider responsibilities, there is a requirement for each of these to cooperate on areas where risk factors may overlap, e.g. clinical or technical staff informing a provider about faulty equipment and the need for a replacement. It is also important to ensure the views of the service user and carer are taken account of, as what is deemed low risk to one service user or carer may indeed be a high risk to another.

Where organisations use third-party providers or suppliers to undertake some of their tasks, it is important for clear boundaries to be set in terms of equipment-related risks, and risk assessments. For example, if a therapist prescribes a specific type of equipment for the service user and the third-party provider does not have that exact type in stock and provides an unsuitable alternative in its place, what are the risks involved and who is responsible for managing them? This is an example of some of the issues to be considered.

Carrying out regular risk assessments is one of the main ways to avoid or minimise the likelihood of incidents occurring, when providing equipment.

It is also important to consider risk issues in terms of assessing the consequence of not providing the equipment at all. For example, failing to provide equipment could result in the service user's condition worsening or in their admission to hospital.

31.1　Risk assessments consider the whole environment where equipment is likely to be used, involve consultation with service users, families and carers, and are carried out in accordance with relevant health and safety requirements, including Management of Health and Safety at Work Regulations 1999, which covers:

- the carrying out of suitable and sufficient risk assessments in respect of both employees and non-employees by a competent person
- making arrangements for the monitoring and reviewing of risk assessments
- putting in place arrangements for the planning, organisation, control, monitoring and review of measures to control risks (preventive and protective measures)
- providing employees with information, instruction and training to ensure their competence and understanding of risks and control measures
- cooperation and coordination between different organisations involved in the provision, maintenance and use of the equipment and the delivery of care to individuals.

31.2 The following specific areas are covered by risk assessments, undertaken by clinical and technical staff, and third-party providers and suppliers (where they make provision on behalf of statutory organisations):

- transportation, assembly and installation of equipment
- safe systems of work and the use of equipment
- risks regarding the trial and demonstration of equipment
- risks arising from the home and the environment where the equipment is to be used
- preventive maintenance and inspection of equipment
- adaptations or modifications
- training, information and instruction
- manual handling issues for staff, equipment users and carers
- emergency procedures, e.g. in event of equipment failure or an emergency
- incident reporting process (where, for example, the equipment provision is hosted by one agency, the incident-reporting process is communicated across all stakeholders to ensure lessons are learned)
- record keeping
- the interface and overlap with third-party providers, where applicable.

CODE STANDARD 32

Reviewing Equipment and Equipment Needs

> **OUTCOME**
> As long as the service user is in possession of equipment, and has a requirement for it, it is safe and continues to meet the service user's needs.

Introduction to Code Standard 32

Reviewing equipment to determine whether or not the equipment is still meeting the needs of the service user is as important as assessing the needs in the first place. To undertake such a task for every service user requires careful planning and staffing resources. Where reviews do not take place, this can present a significant risk to service users.

In addition, without a physical check on the equipment, and possibly a replacement, after a certain period of time as recommended by the manufacturers, service users could potentially be put at risk by using unsafe equipment.

There is no better person for informing as to whether or not their needs are being met than the service user, or their carer, as they are using and living with the equipment every day.

It goes without saying that some simple aids to daily living may not require any follow up, but this should be accordingly risk assessed and factored into any assessment guidance.

It is also important to inform the service user and/or their carer about the expected life of the equipment by providing the manufacturer's instructions, for example. It would also be useful to request that the service user informs the equipment provider if they feel their needs are not being met by the equipment provided.

32.1 There are guidelines available setting out the review and reassessment of service users' equipment needs. There is a formal and robust process in place for tracking and monitoring review and reassessment dates; ideally this will be electronic. This requires close working with the equipment provider.

32.2 Where appropriate, services have systematic review programmes for service users in place. The frequency of the reviews should be consistent with the user's needs and associated risks.

32.3 To ensure equipment continues to meet the needs of the service user, planned clinical reviews are offered to those who need one and the frequency of reviews is agreed with the service user, taking into account, where appropriate:

- progression of condition
- physical and social development
- environment where the equipment is being used, and who is using it
- planned transitions or changes to domestic, vocational or social care arrangements.

32.4 There is a systematic, and preferably electronic, process in place for ensuring equipment is reviewed and replaced, where necessary, in accordance with manufacturers' guidance. Information relating to expected equipment life is widely available and communicated, especially where there is high risk associated with it.

32.5 Where equipment is provided directly by third-party providers or suppliers, the manufacturer's instructions are issued to the service user and/or their carer, as appropriate.

32.6 There is a process and procedure in place for ensuring the service user and/or their family or carer can easily relay their concerns, or self-refer, in the event that the equipment is no longer meeting their needs. This could include supplying a contact telephone number and email address to report any problems.

32.7 There is an agreed hierarchy of review based on equipment types and clinical risk. This will also factor in such things as maintenance requirements and frequency. Manufacturers and suppliers have input into this process to ensure it is in line with their guidance.

32.8 Where alternative options for funding and receiving equipment outside of the normal channels are offered, for example direct payment, personal budgets or vouchers (for wheelchairs), service users and/or their carers are made aware of the need to adhere to manufacturer's recommended period for safe use, and what they should do in the event that the equipment discontinues to meet their needs.

CODE STANDARD 33

Trusted Assessor

OUTCOME

Assessments for simple aids to daily living are carried out by competent individuals.

Introduction to Code Standard 33

Increase in demand for equipment, largely owing to the growing elderly population, has caused many local areas to experience a shortage of professional staff to carry out assessments. This results in delays in assessments and equipment provision, and long waiting lists can ensue. To combat this, some areas use support workers to undertake assessments for simple aids to daily living, instead of fully qualified therapists and nurses. This approach is to be encouraged as a measure of reducing delays in provision, but steps should be taken to ensure the support workers have the necessary skills for this responsible undertaking.

The Trusted Assessor Project (Winchcombe, M. and Ballinger, C. (2005). *A Competence Framework for Trusted Assessors*) was developed to provide support staff with the competencies to safely assess for basic equipment needs.

Some organisations also run in-house training programmes for staff. Whilst these may be as effective as Trusted Assessor training, they may not be linked to any external accreditation.

Where third-party providers or suppliers are used to deliver services on behalf of statutory agencies, it is important to ensure that they are appropriately trained and that the training they receive is delivered by someone competent to do so. Trusted Assessor programmes are ideal for this.

This Code Standard covers Trusted Assessor training as well as training programmes developed in-house, and includes staff of third-party providers and suppliers.

33.1   There is formally recognised and approved Trusted Assessor, or in-house, training provided in the assessment, use and fitting of basic daily living equipment, for all staff who are expected to carry out assessments, but who have not qualified with a professional body.

33.2   Trusted Assessor and in-house training programmes, including training provided to third-party providers or suppliers, are only carried out by a competent person.

33.3   Trusted Assessor training programmes are formally accredited.

33.4   A central database exists with up-to-date training details of all Trusted Assessors, or staff members trained by a competent person, along with other staff who have been identified through performance review to have competencies based on experience to carry out designated assessor duties.

33.5   Regular and ongoing training arrangements are in place for Trusted Assessor or in-house training, or training provided to third-party providers or suppliers, in order to keep up to date with changes in service provision.

33.6   There are clearly defined learning outcomes in place where Trusted Assessor or suitable in-house training is provided.

CODE STANDARD 34

Self-assessment for Equipment

> **OUTCOME**
> Where self-assessment for equipment is offered, there is clear guidance around eligibility, processes, roles, responsibilities and accountability.

Introduction to Code Standard 34

Some authorities offer the opportunity for people to self-assess their needs, generally for simple aids to daily living, or minor adaptations. It is recognised that this equipment or small adaptations to their home, can help people be more independent, and with the right tools, safeguards and support in place, people may be able to assess their own needs.

Where self-assessment is offered, it is important to note that this is not a 'cop-out' in terms of responsibilities. A self-assessment is in addition to, but cannot replace or displace, the local authority's community care assessment. If anything, there need to be more rigorous procedures in place, in view of the following:

- the service user may require several pieces of equipment, some of which may be complex, and these may need to be delivered simultaneously
- equipment may require ongoing maintenance

- equipment may require replacement every so often, according to manufacturers' guidance
- the service user may not be able to collect, install or dispose of equipment due to their disability or illness.

34.1 Where self-assessment is offered, proper safeguards and monitoring arrangements are in place to ensure the service user is:

- given the right equipment
- provided with a safe service
- clear about liability and accountability issues
- offered support to complete the necessary forms, and use online tools, where appropriate.

CODE STANDARD 35

Managing Equipment Budgets

OUTCOME
Resources are managed effectively through clear financial and budgetary authorisation processes and controls.

Introduction to Code Standard 35

Quite often, clinical staff, particularly if they manage the equipment service, will be responsible both for managing equipment budgets, and/or authorising individual items of expenditure for certain pieces of equipment. Without clear financial and budgetary controls in place for staff ordering equipment, overspends can occur; this can lead to delays in equipment provision, or even inability to provide equipment at all, because of a lack of funds.

To manage budgets effectively, it is important that budgets allocated by commissioning authorities bear some relation to both current and future activity within the services, as a shortfall will inevitably put pressure on provision.

Pressure can also arise from service users expecting equipment beyond what the eligibility criteria set by the commissioners will allow them to provide. This also needs to be well managed.

Furthermore, the introduction and availability of alternative funding options, e.g. direct payments, personal budgets or vouchers, can add significant pressure to funding and budgets, if not well managed. Where funding is allocated to the service user to purchase equipment, in most cases the equipment will belong to the service user and will not be recycled. This can prove to be a more costly method of provision.

It is good practice for clinical staff to have awareness of budgetary constraints, and of what equipment is held in store before ordering new, as this information will help with managing the budget.

35.1 Where budgetary responsibilities for managing or controlling equipment spend are given to clinical staff, via a scheme of financial delegation or otherwise, clear responsibilities are set out in terms of their budget allocations, and the conditions of expenditure, e.g. thresholds and authorisation levels.

35.2 Budgetary responsibilities for managing or controlling equipment spend are bound by the financial frameworks, e.g. standing orders, and procurement regulations of the employing organisations.

35.3 Those with responsibility for managing or controlling equipment spend have access to, and are able to provide, expenditure reports, including committed and projected spend, for example.

35.4 Processes exist to demonstrate how those with responsibility for managing or controlling equipment spend ensure the most efficient practice and best value is achieved when ordering new equipment.

PART FOUR

PERIPHERAL ISSUES AND SPECIALIST AREAS

Introduction to Code Standards 36 to 47

Part 4 is a supplementary section, covering 'non-standard' areas which may or may not be relevant. Organisations or individuals working to Parts 1, 2, and 3 of the Code should also work to individual Code Standards from Part 4, which are relevant to their activities.

If not well managed, peripheral aspects of service provision, such as cross-border issues, and alternative funding arrangements like personal budgets and vouchers (for wheelchairs), for example, can present complications. Failure to address these issues adequately, and have the necessary safeguards in place, can expose service users to risk, and a lack of clear decision making results in significant delays in equipment provision.

Although most equipment provided by the public sector is issued via a local equipment service, there are a significant number of other sources of statutory provision, e.g. equipment in schools, continuing healthcare equipment. External suppliers and providers are also commissioned to provide some or all aspects of service provision.

Generally these periphery areas of service provision are overlooked and neglected, and there are few clear boundaries in terms of responsibilities and accountabilities, for equipment from these sources. This poses risks to service users, especially if, for example, servicing and maintenance of equipment provided outside of standard equipment services, falls outside of anyone's attention.

Involvement of service users and carers is often held up as good practice; but sadly this rich source of input is not widely embraced, and where it is, involvement is often too late to be beneficial. The involvement of service users and their carers is just as important, if not more, than any other aspect of the overall commissioning and provider functions. It should therefore be viewed as a core element, not as a 'periphery' aspect.

This Part contains Code Standards aimed at addressing and managing various aspects of equipment provision that are often overlooked.

Note

Parts 1–3 of this Code of Practice may also have application to organisations providing equipment in a specialist service area, e.g. schools, even if provision is not made through a statutory equipment service. For example, equipment in schools is subject to the same health and safety requirements as an equipment service, and must be properly commissioned. This Part does not restate relevant requirements already set down in earlier sections; it gives additional requirements relevant specifically to the following specialist areas of provision.

CODE STANDARD 36

Equipment in Special Schools

> **OUTCOME**
> Equipment is provided safely and continues to meet the individual needs of service users.

Introduction to Code Standard 36

Although this Code Standard has been developed particularly with special schools in mind, the principles also apply where equipment is provided in any educational setting.

The provision of equipment in special schools is generally considered to be problematic. Poor wheelchair accessibility is a common problem, in particular. Special schools often lack the appropriate facilities and resources to manage all aspects of equipment, e.g. access, maintenance and decontamination, safely and effectively.

Although there are various plans and arrangements in place for trying to address the provision of equipment for children in schools, provision largely operates as a standalone service; this is partly because of the different funding and commissioning arrangements across health, social care and education. There are significant benefits in being able to jointly fund and share equipment, both inside and outside of the school. Doing so also offers a more person-centred and holistic service to children and their families. Following some of the other Code Standards for commissioning, as set out in Part 1, could pave the way for an integrated and seamless approach.

Workable solutions should be sought to allow people to use life-enhancing equipment everywhere they need to, and schools should be no exception.

36.1 There is evidence that equipment provided in schools is subject to all relevant health and safety obligations and medical devices regulations.

36.2 Equipment is electronically recorded, traceable, and is subject to planned maintenance scheduling arrangements.

36.3 Formal commissioning/contracting arrangements exist for the provision of equipment in schools and, where appropriate, across a range of settings.

36.4 There is an allocated budget, or pooled budgets/joint funding, for the provision of disability equipment in schools. Note this may also include alternative funding options.

36.5 There are protocols in place for arranging and funding a range of assistive technologies, e.g. communication equipment, to meet all the needs of the service user.

36.6 Efforts are made to ensure equipment can be shared outside the school environment, e.g. at home, where appropriate.

36.7 All staff involved in the assessment, provision and maintenance of equipment are appropriately trained and competent to do so.

CODE STANDARD 37

Complex, Specialist and Children's Equipment

> **OUTCOME**
> Service users requiring complex, specialist or children's equipment are assessed appropriately, and provided with suitable equipment in a safe and timely manner.

Introduction to Code Standard 37

The provision of complex, specialist and children's equipment is commonly recognised as being difficult to manage, in many aspects. There are often delays with these types of equipment. This can be owing to poor commissioning, inadequate eligibility criteria, funding, assessments and provision.

This equipment includes complex wheelchairs, children's postural support equipment, bariatric beds, communication aids and sensory impairment aids – basically all non-standard equipment.

Often these types of equipment are required urgently for people with rapidly progressing conditions or terminal illnesses. In these instances, it is important to arrange for equipment to be fast-tracked and provided as soon as possible.

Poor service provision for people with complex and specialist needs directly impacts upon the lives and wellbeing of many vulnerable individuals right across the health, social care and education spectrum. As an example, failing to get the right postural support equipment for children in a timely way can result in long-term developmental implications.

Limiting provision of complex, specialist and children's equipment, or not providing it in a timely way, can often be much more costly in the longer term by leading to secondary, and unnecessary, episodes of care. Some common issues arising from poor provision include:

- unacceptable quality leading to unnecessary episodes of care, e.g. hospitalisation, admission to care homes
- a loss of access to schools, and impaired length and quality of life (children)
- exposure to litigation and prosecution for non-compliance with civil and criminal legislation
- services being unnecessarily costly and unsustainable, by failing to exploit scale economies, collaboration or sharing of resource.

It should now be easier to address this difficult area as there is a greater drive to promote integrated and joint working between health, social care, housing and education agencies.

37.1   There are formal and suitable arrangements in place for dealing with all aspects of complex, specialist and children's equipment, including:

- commissioning and contracting, including joint working
- funding, including alternative funding options, e.g. personal budgets, vouchers
- publicly available eligibility criteria
- fast-tracking arrangements for people with rapidly progressing conditions and terminal illnesses, for example
- operational issues, including purchasing, storage, decontamination, medical device management, planned maintenance scheduling, health and safety, delivery, and risk management
- training for staff in assessments, use of and repair of equipment.

37.2 A specialist assessment is available for those with complex or specialist needs, particularly for wheelchair and seating needs, and this aims to be person-centred, anticipatory and conducted in the context of a multidisciplinary team. The following aspects of special assessments are also considered:

- robust screening and prioritising process
- following evidence-based good practice guidelines
- undertaken by competent, registered clinical staff with specialist knowledge and skills
- managed collaboratively by relevant care services using case management approaches.

CODE STANDARD 38

Continuing Healthcare Equipment

> **OUTCOME**
> Equipment provided for continuing healthcare needs is safe, suitable, and is covered by appropriate maintenance and breakdown arrangements.

Introduction to Code Standard 38

Continuing healthcare is a general term describing the care that children and adults need, over an extended period of time as a result of illness, accident or disability. It can address both physical and mental health needs.

Continuing healthcare can be provided in a range of settings, such as a hospital, a registered care home or a person's own home. The types of health care services provided include primary health care, respite health care, community health services, and health care equipment. The responsibility for provision of care and equipment lies with the NHS.

A person considered to be eligible for continuing healthcare will generally have: complex health care needs, and/or intensive health care needs, and/or unstable/unpredictable health care needs; rapid deterioration. Qualifying individuals will also require significant health care inputs, such as regular supervision by a member of the NHS care team, e.g. a therapist, and routine use of specialist health care equipment.

The difficulty with the equipment provided for continuing healthcare service users is that it is quite often very specialist, e.g. a ventilator. The equipment therefore requires rigorous safety checks and support. However, because this type of equipment does not usually go through the usual equipment service route, the maintenance and support is often provided directly by suppliers, if at all. This means that equipment responsibilities, e.g. planned maintenance schedules, can sometimes be overlooked, and in some cases completely ignored. This is a huge risk to the service user as some of this equipment is life supporting, and to the responsible organisation in terms of risk and accountability.

In some areas people may obtain their equipment by the use of alternative funding options, e.g. personal health budgets; again this poses significant risk where the necessary safeguards are not built into the process, including maintenance and ongoing support.

38.1   There are formal and suitable arrangements in place for dealing with all aspects of continuing healthcare equipment, including:

- commissioning and contracting
- funding (whole-life costs, e.g. maintenance, calibration, specialist decontamination)
- operational issues, including purchasing, storage, decontamination, medical device management, planned maintenance scheduling, health and safety, delivery, and training for staff in use of and repair of equipment
- the ability to recall equipment if necessary.

38.2   Where equipment is ordered directly from the supplier, to go to a service user's home, there are suitable medical device management arrangements in place, including all aspects of maintenance and breakdown cover. This is supported by an in-house database showing where equipment is, and when it next requires maintenance.

38.3   Any equipment ordered has the approval of medical device management boards, or similar in-house technical authority.

38.4   Service users are provided with user instructions, together with information outlining what to do in the event of product failure, or failure of ancillary supplies needed for the equipment to function, for example.

38.5   Where alternative funding for equipment has been granted, e.g. personal health budgets, information outlining responsibilities is made available and communicated to the service user.

CODE STANDARD 39

Equipment in Care Homes

> **OUTCOME**
> There is clarity around the roles, responsibilities, obligations and legal requirements where equipment is provided into a care home.

Introduction to Code Standard 39

This Code Standard specifically relates to where equipment is provided into a care home by another organisation, and the obligations and considerations for each respective party.

There is often a lack of clarity in terms of roles, responsibilities and obligations when equipment is provided into care homes (nursing and residential). Consequently some local areas develop their own protocol for equipment going into care homes. Whatever the approach, legal responsibilities must be made clear, e.g. health and safety, medical device management.

Where an equipment service provides equipment into a care home the service should still expect to meet all relevant health and safety, and medical device management responsibilities, e.g. planned maintenance and repairs, unless formal arrangements have been put in place to transfer those responsibilities to the care home.

Even without a transfer of responsibilities, the care home should be responsible for cleaning the equipment regularly, whilst in use, and complying with relevant manufacturer's instructions for the equipment, whilst in use.

Where a resident brings their own equipment into a residential care setting, there are issues relating to suitability and maintenance, for example, which should be considered.

39.1   Where equipment is provided by organisations into care homes there is a clear protocol setting out roles and responsibilities for both parties. Care homes are made aware of this protocol, before its introduction. The protocol includes, but is not limited to:

- cleaning responsibilities (whilst in use)
- planned maintenance responsibilities, e.g. LOLER testing
- emergency breakdown cover, including out of hours
- guidance on following manufacturer's instructions
- contact details.

39.2   There is a list available of equipment types and eligibility criteria for equipment provision into care homes, for relevant staff and organisations to refer to.

39.3   Terms and conditions are agreed before equipment is issued into the care home. If agreeable, care homes sign this, either upon receipt of equipment or as part of an overall contract. This specifies the responsibilities of both parties, and the conditions which must be met before equipment can be issued. It includes, for example, acknowledgement that:

- all pieces of equipment remain the property of the equipment service or providing organisation at all times
- the pieces of equipment received are for the sole use of the patient named on the requisition for equipment
- the care home will advise the equipment service or providing organisation when the resident no longer has need of the equipment

- the care home accepts responsibility for all risks should the equipment be used by any patient other than the person for whom the item was requested
- the care home will pay for any lost items, or any equipment damaged or broken through negligence or misuse.

39.4   Where equipment is brought in to the care home by the resident, a risk assessment is undertaken to look at the suitability of the equipment. Identified risks are discussed with the resident and mutual agreement is reached as to how the risks are to be managed.

CODE STANDARD 40

Hospital Discharge Arrangements

> **OUTCOME**
> Provision of necessary equipment is a seamless part of hospital discharge.

Introduction to Code Standard 40

There are many equipment-related reasons for hospital discharges being delayed, for example:

- delayed and problematic service user requirements and home assessments
- arranging suitable times and dates, etc. for equipment to be delivered and/or installed in the service user's home
- adaptations, complex, specialist and/or children's equipment are required, which take time to acquire
- complex packages of care involving different health and social care agencies
- equipment package provided from different sources
- cross-border difficulties, i.e. discharging a service user into a different county/local authority boundary
- poor communication and formal arrangements between hospital and community-based staff
- funding issues.

Whatever the reason for delays, it is clearly important to ensure robust and streamlined systems and procedures exist to minimise delays. It is also important to ensure that whatever procedures are used, these are widely communicated and understood.

Where equipment is required urgently, for terminally ill people, for example, there is opportunity for organisations working in collaboration with other strategic partners, e.g. third sector organisations, to ensure some equipment can be provided quickly, and to facilitate a prompt hospital discharge.

40.1 Both hospital and community-based staff work to mutually agreed hospital discharge assessment and access criteria to manage service users both with temporary impairment and chronic, permanent conditions.

40.2 There are fast-tracking arrangements in place, and included in hospital discharge procedures, to ensure people with rapidly progressing conditions and terminal illnesses can access routine and complex equipment urgently.

40.3 Hospital staff responsible for discharging service users are trained in both the assessment and the provision aspects of equipment.

40.4 Where service users require equipment to facilitate a hospital discharge, the process is reflected within a mutually agreed policy between hospital and community-based health and social care organisations. This includes a communication plan with community staff, and also equipment services. This reflects the operational functions of the equipment services, e.g. contact details, opening hours, delivery schedules. It also includes cross-border arrangements, and links with different agencies.

40.5 Where third-party providers or suppliers are used as part of core provision, there is a protocol demonstrating the ordering and delivery processes where a service user needs equipment from different sources to enable a safe hospital discharge. This links to the hospital discharge policy.

CODE STANDARD 41

Alternative Funding Options for Equipment

OUTCOME
Anyone obtaining equipment via an alternative payment route will do so in a straightforward and timely manner; they will also be given clear guidance relating to ownership responsibilities, including breakdown, maintenance and disposal.

Introduction to Code Standard 41

Some organisations offer alternative funding options to enable service users to purchase equipment themselves. These payment options may come under a range of names including, for example, a direct payment, a personal budget, a personal health budget, an integrated budget, an individual budget, or a voucher via the voucher scheme (used for acquiring wheelchairs). These options are offered generally with the view to providing the service user with more choice, flexibility and control over their own care.

One of the potential advantages with alternative funding options is that individuals may choose to buy their equipment from a different supplier or provider to the one the statutory organisation uses, where they can put the money towards a more costly, highly specified model that they feel meets their needs better.

Service users do not have to receive an alternative funding option if they prefer the statutory organisation to provide the equipment for them.

Generally speaking, equipment obtained using an alternative funding option will belong to the service user, unless there is some form of partnership agreement in place between the awarding organisation and the service user (or someone acting on their behalf). The service user will generally be responsible for its care and maintenance – although discretionary rules can apply relating to ownership and maintenance to reflect the best interest of the service user. Also, in some instances additional sums of money may be added to the initial payment to cover a warranty, as well as ongoing maintenance, etc.

Where any of the alternative funding options are given to the service user to acquire their own equipment, it is most important that safeguards are in place to allow this to happen safely, as set out below.

41.1   Organisations offering alternative funding options have a clear policy and procedure in place for staff and potential service users to be able to access.

41.2   Organisations offering alternative funding options have a user agreement in place which clearly sets out how the funding should be used. Information within an agreement includes, but is not excluded to: names and addresses, conditions of the agreement, payment arrangements and user's contribution, proof of sale, warranty, review details, maintenance, ownership and disposal.

41.3   Where an alternative funding option is provided, risk and safety issues are included in the agreement.

41.4   Where alternative funding options for equipment are granted, conditions for accessing more funds for equipment are clearly communicated to the service user to cover such things as changing health needs and when equipment is no longer fit for purpose.

CODE STANDARD 42

Establishing Links between Assistive Technology-related Services

---

OUTCOME

Organisations communicate effectively and collaborate formally with other assistive technology-related services, to reduce delays and duplication for service users.

Introduction to Code Standard 42

Quite often similar assistive technology-related services, e.g. wheelchair services, community equipment services, telecare services and speech and language departments, provide separate services to the same service user. This can result in separate assessments and equipment provision, involving duplication in time, cost and effort. Similarly, there are cases where different clinical professionals, e.g. occupational therapists, community nurses and physiotherapists, make separate assessments for the same service user. Having several assessments and several deliveries of equipment, arriving at different times, can be disconcerting for the service user, and are a poor use of resource in terms of the clinical professionals' time.

In addition, equipment-related data and information for the different assistive technology-related services are generally held separately. As a result of this, there is no central database recording all the equipment and assistive technologies a service user has been provided with. This makes it difficult to look at the total equipment care package collectively and to determine whether or not the holistic needs of the service user have been met.

These difficulties may also be compounded in regions where third-party providers and suppliers are also used to support statutory provision.

For there to be any real 'integration' and closer and established links with other strategic assistive technology-related partners, including a joint approach to assessments and data sharing, there needs to be formal agreement at a commissioning and organisational level.

42.1 The strategy for services and/or the service specification for the provision of equipment services include links between associated services, e.g. communication aids, telecare, outlining how services will work in collaboration to ensure duplication is minimised, and that services are provided as efficiently and timely as possible.

42.2 Equipment services establish formal links with related equipment providers to ensure that critical life-change transitions affecting service users and/or carers (child to adult service user, loss of key carer, e.g. parent, and university to workplace) are seamless and coordinated, with input from the service user and carer.

42.3 Suitable arrangements are in place to ensure assessments and equipment deliveries are minimised to reduce the number of contacts experienced by the service user.

42.4 Where services are working jointly there is a database, or cross-reference data available, in an accessible format, to ensure clinical professionals can view all the equipment possessed by service users.

42.5 Where third-party providers or suppliers are used to support statutory provision, information is available to show what equipment the service user has.

42.6 There is a clear communication plan in place to ensure equipment care packages coming from different sources, e.g. equipment stores and third-party providers, are coordinated.

CODE STANDARD 43

Third-party Contractors

> **OUTCOME**
> All third-party contractors have their quality and performance-related requirements clearly communicated and documented, and these are closely monitored and reviewed on a regular basis.

Introduction to Code Standard 43

It is common for some aspects of equipment services to be provided by third-party contractors and suppliers, including retailers. This may be the provision of logistics, repairs or decontamination processes, for example; in some cases a significant part of the equipment service may be provided by a third party. In these cases it is still important to ensure that all legal obligations are being met, as outsourcing parts of service provision does not in any way reduce statutory duties and responsibilities.

It is important, therefore, that no matter what aspects are undertaken by third-party providers, responsibilities are clearly set out from the beginning, and there are measures in place for ensuring that those responsibilities are being met.

43.1 Where components of equipment services are outsourced to third-party contractors, this is formally and mutually agreed, as appropriate, e.g. contract, service level agreement, memorandum of understanding.

43.2   Third-party service providers have been made aware of the legal responsibilities they are expected to meet. This is in place prior to contract award, or commissioning of service provision, and is mutually agreed.

43.3   Where third-party services are operating they are subject to the same contract management processes as in-house providers, e.g. quality and performance management reports, together with relevant key performance indicator compliance, as appropriate.

43.4   Staff employed by third-party providers are subject to the same requirements as in-house services, e.g. training.

CODE STANDARD 44

Outsourced Service Providers

> **OUTCOME**
> Where services are fully outsourced, all contractual, liability, accountability, quality and performance-related issues are mutually agreed and clearly documented.

Introduction to Code Standard 44

Some equipment services are fully outsourced to external providers, as an alternative way of providing services. This approach is sometimes viewed as passing responsibility from the statutory authority to the external provider. This is only partly true as the ultimate responsibility for ensuring service users get a satisfactory service, and that their needs are being met, still lies with the statutory authority.

In some cases it makes good commercial sense to outsource provision, as the external providers may be able to run the service more efficiently, for example, by being able to generate economies of scale by operating nationally.

Regardless of how services are provided, it ultimately remains the responsibility of the commissioners, or those responsible for purchasing services, to ensure that what they are expecting the external provider to do has been clearly stipulated, mutually agreed upon and formally contracted, including a service specification, for example.

44.1   Those responsible for commissioning and purchasing services ensure that what they are expecting the external provider to do has been clearly stipulated, mutually agreed upon and formally contracted, including a clear service specification, for example.

44.2   Outsourced services are subject to the same provider responsibilities as in-house providers, including (where appropriate):

- involvement of users and carers
- operational management
- quality management systems
- training and qualifications
- information technology and information management
- health and safety management
- transportation
- decontamination
- performance management
- emergency and out-of-hours cover
- stock management
- recycling
- assembling, fitting and demonstrating equipment
- minor adaptations
- manual handling
- medical device management.

44.3   Where outsourced service provision includes clinical responsibilities, these are subject to the same responsibilities as in-house clinical staff, including, for example:

- assessing and reviewing the service user's equipment needs
- training in equipment provision and use
- equipment selection process
- demonstrating and trialling equipment
- risk assessments.

CODE STANDARD 45

Involvement of Service Users and Carers

> **OUTCOME**
> The planning, design, commissioning, procurement, performance
> standards, product selection of equipment, and review of services,
> involves service users and/or carers as a matter of course.

Introduction to Code Standard 45

The commissioning and provision of equipment services is ultimately to assist
and support clinical teams and organisations in the delivery of appropriate care
to service users. It is therefore important that the views of users, and their
carers, are taken into account when planning, designing or reviewing service
provision. Views may be captured by directly involving users and carers on
various groups, or by gaining feedback through questionnaires, for example.

The involvement of service users and carers in the development of
equipment services is crucial. They can make a contribution at several levels.
As individuals they can contribute from their own experience of using the
services. This information may be gathered during the assessment process,
at the review stage or via some form of survey.

Service users and carers can also contribute by being involved in the
planning and development of the service through representation on the
various forums charged with developing services.

45.1 There is evidence that commissioners/planning teams, providers and clinical teams have taken input from service users and/or carers when developing services, strategies and policies. Some example roles and responsibilities of service users include:

- input into the planning and development of relevant policies and strategies
- interpreting policy into service delivery
- reviews of assessment facilities and new equipment
- review of outcomes from questionnaires and surveys, etc.
- analysing and reviewing compliments and complaints
- advising on local and national disability policies and/or legislation.

45.2 Where appropriate, service users and/or carers are actively informed and involved in the development of equipment specifications, the equipment review and selection processes, and in a formal feedback process about the overall satisfaction with service provision. Feedback is gathered through the use of various means, e.g. social media platforms.

45.3 Service users and their carers are treated as equal partners in planning, developing and assessing care to make sure it is most appropriate for their needs and they are at the heart of all decisions. This is in keeping with the person-centred care agenda.

45.4 Where alternative funding options are granted as a means of acquiring equipment, views are sought from service users both before and after the funds have been awarded to ensure their needs are, and continue to be, met satisfactorily.

CODE STANDARD 46

Cross-border Protocol

OUTCOME
Suitable arrangements exist to ensure service users who require equipment and who are affected by geographical boundaries have their equipment needs met in a safe, coordinated and timely manner.

Introduction to Code Standard 46

Cross-border issues can be very problematic when providing equipment, especially where there are no clear guidelines about geographical areas of responsibility. Problems arising from this issue impact upon many areas of care, where equipment is required. Some examples of these include:

- hospital discharges
- disabled children and young people in special schools, children's homes or in foster care
- residential and nursing homes
- respite care
- service users moving home.

46.1 There is a local cross-border protocol in existence outlining the following areas of responsibility:

- the geographical area where equipment will be provided
- funding and recharging for out-of-county arrangements
- service responsibilities for county residents outside the county, e.g. at university, special schools
- residential and nursing home provision
- communication protocol
- process for making referrals
- relevant contact details for equipment providers, including opening hours, for example
- the types of equipment that will be provided by the various services.

CODE STANDARD 47

Disabled Facilities Grants (DFGs) and Major Adaptations

> **OUTCOME**
> Service users requiring major adaptations and a Disabled Facilities Grant are assessed appropriately, and provided with suitable equipment in a safe, coordinated and timely manner.

Introduction to Code Standard 47

A Disabled Facilities Grant (DFG) is a means-tested grant designed to help meet the costs of adaptations to a property for a disabled occupant. In order to qualify for a DFG, the required adaptations need to be considered *necessary and appropriate* (by the housing department, but on a recommendation by social services) to meet the needs of the disabled person, and it must be considered *reasonable and practicable* (by the housing department) for the relevant works to be carried out.

Disabled Facilities Grants must be given to provide facilities deemed necessary and appropriate to meet the needs of the disabled person.

Some of the types of work carried out under a DFG include: have easier access to and from the property; have easier access to a room used or that can be used as a bedroom; have easier access to a room in which there is a toilet, bath or shower. Major adaptations are usually in excess of £1,000, and can be anywhere up to £30,000 in value; they include, for example: ramps, stairlifts, vertical lifts, door widening, level access shower, overhead ceiling track hoists. The maximum award currently for a DFG is £30,000. As this grant is means-tested, some people may have to pay a contribution towards the required work themselves. However, local housing authorities have discretion, but not a duty, to exceed the £30,000 amount.

There is often ambiguity surrounding certain aspects of major adaptation provision, for example, who has responsibility for funding certain aspects of works, supplier contracts and ongoing maintenance?

One of the main criticisms of DFGs is the length of time it takes from referral through to approval. In some cases this can be up to two years. Some of the reasons for these delays include: service users' availability, property ownership, financial resources, landlords' consent, building regulations approval, and obtaining detailed quotations for the agreed works.

Local authorities are required to provide an answer to an application for a DFG as soon as is reasonably practicable, and no later than six months after the application is made. The actual payment of the DFG should take place no more than twelve months after the application was made.

Local authorities have a duty to try to reduce any problems or suffering caused by the lack of suitable accommodation while a DFG is being considered. This can include providing funding for a temporary move to more suitable accommodation.

47.1   An efficient, consistent and timely adaptations service is provided.

47.2   A range of major adaptations are on offer to assist service users to remain safe and comfortable, and to maintain their independence within their own homes.

47.3   Assistance is given to those in need of adaptations to make informed choices about their housing options, facilitating transfers to more appropriate accommodation where required.

47.4   The adaptations required are considered along with the service user's priority. Prioritisation is based on the needs of the individual, any existing health and safety risks to the individual and/or their carer, and takes into account rapidly progressive conditions or terminal illnesses.

47.5   Assistance is offered to households whose current home is unsuitable for major adaptations. Where only extensive, costly adaptations will meet the particular needs of a household, rehousing options are considered.

47.6   All adaptation work completed on a housing association owned property is recorded to ensure future allocations of the property are made to applicants requiring such adaptations, wherever practicable.

47.7   Contractors carrying out adaptations are closely monitored by those with the right technical skills to ensure the work meets the required standard, complies with the occupational therapist's original recommendation and takes the service user's needs into account.

47.8   There is clarity around the responsibility for the servicing and ongoing maintenance of all adaptations.

47.9   Service users are kept informed about the progress of their DFG and adaptation, and their views are sought on their satisfaction with completed works.

47.10   The DFG policy is reviewed on a regular basis in line with legislative or regulatory changes.

47.11   Where an adaptation is required, a process seeking formal agreement is followed. This may include the service user, carer, other members of the household, and other appropriate agencies.

APPENDICES

Appendix 1
Legislation relating to disability equipment in the UK

Appendix 2
Guide for contract management indicators

Appendix 3
Semta Occupational Standards specifically for equipment technicians

Appendix 4
Supporting guidance relating to training on Information Systems and Information Management for individual roles

Appendix 5
Supporting guidance relating to Medical Device Management

Appendix 6
Supporting guidance relating to the choice of decontamination method appropriate to the degree of infection risk associated with the intended use of the equipment

Appendix 7
Glossary

Appendix 1

Legislation relating to disability equipment in the UK

The following list highlights some of the main pieces of legislation with relevance to disability equipment services. It is for guidance only and is by no means exhaustive.

Note that health and welfare-related legislation and specific regulatory obligations have not been included in this appendix as these are subject to regular change, and are sometimes different across the countries of the UK. It is strongly recommended that individuals and organisations keep up to date with relevant legislation in the region which they operate in, and to seek the advice of legal departments within their own organisation.

Each piece of legislation listed below is explained further in the remainder of this appendix, where its relevance to disability equipment is discussed, and areas where the requirements could be breached are highlighted in the shaded boxes.

UN Convention on the Rights of Disabled People
UN Convention on the Rights of the Child (UNCRC)
Corporate Manslaughter and Corporate Homicide Act 2007
**Human Rights Act 1998 (European Convention on Human
    Rights)**
Health and Safety at Work etc. Act 1974
Management of Health and Safety at Work Regulations 1999
The Health and Safety (Offences) Act 2008
Common Law of Negligence
Consumer Protection Act 1987 (Part 1)
General Product Safety Regulations 2005
Manual Handling Operations Regulations 1992

Medical Devices Regulations 2002 (Amended 2003)

Sale and Supply of Goods and Services Act 1982 and Sale and
 Supply of Goods Act 1994

MHRA Managing Medical Devices DB2006 (05) November 2006

Lifting Operations and Lifting Equipment Regulations 1998
 (LOLER)

Provision and Use of Work Equipment Regulations 1998
 (PUWER)

Control of Substances Hazardous to Health Regulations 2002
 (COSHH)

The Reporting of Injuries, Diseases and Dangerous Occurrences
 Regulations 1995 (RIDDOR)

UN Convention on the Rights of Disabled People

Note. This Convention is known as The Rights of Persons with Disabilities in
other parts of the United Nations. The Office for Disability Issues chose to
retitle it for use in the UK.

The main purpose of the Convention is to promote, protect and ensure the
full and equal enjoyment of all human rights and fundamental freedoms by
all persons with disabilities, and to promote respect for their inherent
dignity.

It is a requirement for public sector organisations, including equipment
providers, to ensure their service provision reflects and includes:
participation and inclusion, non-discrimination, accessibility, personal
mobility and rehabilitation issues, as set out in the Convention.

POTENTIAL LEGAL BREACHES

Failing to provide a service to certain service user groups would
most certainly breach the Convention rules, e.g. children requiring
equipment to access the education system.

Failing to provide equipment to certain service user groups whose

---

> needs have been assessed, but are not provided with equipment, particularly when the need fits within the eligibility criteria, could also be in breach of the Convention.

UN Convention on the Rights of the Child (UNCRC)

This UN Convention is an international human rights treaty that applies to all children and young people aged eighteen and under. It is the most widely ratified international human rights instrument and gives children and young people a wide range of civil, political, economic, social and cultural rights which State Parties to the Convention are expected to implement.

Article 23 contains sections with particular relevance to disability equipment provision, as follows:

1. State Parties recognize that a mentally or physically disabled child should enjoy a full and decent life, in conditions which ensure dignity, promote self-reliance and facilitate the child's active participation in the community.

2. State Parties recognize the right of the disabled child to special care and shall encourage and ensure the extension, subject to available resources, to the eligible child and those responsible for his or her care, of assistance for which application is made and which is appropriate to the child's condition and to the circumstances of the parents or others caring for the child.

3. Recognizing the special needs of a disabled child, assistance extended in accordance with paragraph two of the present article shall be provided free of charge, whenever possible, taking into account the financial resources of the parents or others caring for the child, and shall be designed to ensure that the disabled child has effective access to and receives education, training, health care services, rehabilitation services, preparation for employment and recreation opportunities in a manner conducive to the child's achieving the fullest possible social

integration and individual development, including his or her cultural and spiritual development.

4.   State Parties shall promote, in the spirit of international cooperation, the exchange of appropriate information in the field of preventive health care and of medical, psychological and functional treatment of disabled children, including dissemination of and access to information concerning methods of rehabilitation, education and vocational services, with the aim of enabling State Parties to improve their capabilities and skills and to widen their experience in these areas. In this regard, particular account shall be taken of the needs of developing countries.

POTENTIAL LEGAL BREACHES
Failing to provide necessary equipment and support to children and their carers might be considered to be in breach of the Convention. Failure also to ensure eligibility criteria is in keeping with the requirements of the Convention, and article 23 in particular, may also be considered as a breach of the Convention.

Corporate Manslaughter and Corporate Homicide Act 2007

In summary, an organisation is guilty of corporate manslaughter if the way in which its activities are managed or organised causes a death and amounts to a gross breach of a relevant duty of care to the deceased. A substantial part of the breach must have been in the way activities were managed by senior management, which could be either commissioners or provider management.

The offence is particularly concerned with organisations, including partnerships. Individuals can still be prosecuted separately for health and safety negligence by, for example, the Health and Safety Executive, and by the Crown Prosecution Service for gross negligence manslaughter in common law.

The law therefore allows for collective decisions like, for example, partnership board decisions.

For the offence to apply, an organisation must have owed a 'relevant duty of care' to the victim. The Act defines a duty of care as '…an obligation that an organisation has to take reasonable steps to protect a person's safety'. This includes, for example, equipment used by employees, systems of work, products and services supplied to customers – or in this case, service users.

Some of the 'duties' outlined within section two of the Act are connected to: supplying goods and services; commercial activities; construction and maintenance work; using or keeping plant, and vehicles. All of these could be relevant to the day-to-day activities carried out by equipment services.

POTENTIAL LEGAL BREACHES
The Health and Safety Executive (HSE) writes concerning the Corporate Manslaughter and Corporate Homicide Act that:

'Companies and organisations should keep their health and safety management systems under review, in particular, the way in which their activities are managed and organised by senior management.'

In view of this, a potential breach could be the commissioners of an organisation failing to specify or have any controls in place for managing high risk areas, e.g. not getting equipment maintained to save cost.

This is quite a broad area but the most obvious factors which could potentially lead to a breach are serious failings with: Health and Safety at Work etc. Act 1974, Management of Health and Safety at Work Regulations 1999, and the governance arrangements in place.

Human Rights Act 1998 (European Convention on Human Rights)

This relates more to the decision-making process of the equipment service, from both the commissioner, prescriber and provider of the service. These must ensure that people have the right not to be subjected to 'inhuman or degrading treatment' – see article three for further details.

In addition, article eight outlines the right to respect for home, family and private life.

Article fourteen suggests that there should be freedom from any form of discrimination.

POTENTIAL LEGAL BREACHES

'Discretionary decisions, including omissions to act, i.e. all policy making, practices, procedures, actions, individual decisions, will become potentially challengeable for a breach of human rights.' (www.careandhealthlaw.com – Accessed January 2009)

Where the consequence of not providing a piece of equipment is that the service user would be subjected to inhuman/degrading circumstances, e.g. having to urinate in the living room (assuming the service user has been assessed and is eligible), and a decision is made not to supply, there could in some circumstances be a potential breach of the Act/Convention.

Health and Safety at Work etc. Act 1974

Health and Safety at Work etc. Act 1974, section 2. Employers have a duty to ensure, so far as is reasonably practicable, the health, safety and welfare at work of all their employees.

Duty of employers to non-employees: Health and Safety at Work etc. Act 1974, section 3. Every employer has a duty to conduct its undertaking in such a way as to ensure, so far as is reasonably practicable, that people not in its employment but who may be affected by the undertaking are not thereby exposed to risk to their health and safety.

Section 2 of the Health and Safety at Work etc. Act 1974 looks at the 'General duties of employers to their employees', and includes activities carried out in the community. Section 3 covers users and carers by outlining the 'General duties of employers and self-employed to persons other than their employees'. Basically section 3 states the duty of employers to ensure persons not in their employment are not exposed to risks (so far as is reasonably practicable) to their health and safety, and also it is the responsibility of every employer to provide appropriate information to such individuals about the way undertakings are conducted which might affect their health and safety.

Particular relevance to equipment provision under section 2 and section 3 would include such things as: appropriate acquisition methods, inspecting, checking, recording, tracking, recall, training, maintenance, cleaning, storing, demonstrating, lifting operations, delivering, instructions, repair, replacement, and emergency call-out.

POTENTIAL LEGAL BREACHES
Failure to conduct any of the tasks listed above safely could potentially breach this Act. It is worth noting that there have already been some prosecutions relating to these types of issues, e.g. accidents with hoists, overhead ceiling track hoists, bedrails.

Management of Health and Safety at Work Regulations 1999
The regulations state: 'Every employer shall make a suitable and sufficient assessment of:

(a) the risks to the health and safety of his employees to which they are exposed whilst they are at work; and
(b) the risks to the health and safety of persons not in his employment arising out of or in connection by him of his undertaking.'

The regulations also require all employers, and in this context equipment partners/commissioners, to plan, organise, monitor and review work procedures. This also requires formal assessment of risks, especially where employees and any others might be affected by health and safety failures.

POTENTIAL LEGAL BREACHES

There would be a clear breach of these regulations if there was a serious untoward incident, and it was discovered that there were no written governance arrangements in place, including risk management processes. It is likely that poorly drafted contractual arrangements would also breach the regulations, in the event of an incident.

The Health and Safety (Offences) Act 2008

The Health and Safety (Offences) Act 2008 came into effect on 16 January 2009 and increased the number of circumstances in which employees may be imprisoned for health and safety breaches.

The Act introduced tough new penalties to act as a deterrent to organisations that are tempted to flout the law. Certain offences are now triable in either the Magistrates' Court or the Crown Court. Employees could find themselves at risk of imprisonment under the law if they fail to take reasonable care of the health and safety of others or even themselves. In addition, a director and senior manager can infringe the law where the problem was caused with their consent, connivance or neglect.

POTENTIAL LEGAL BREACHES

Failure to meet existing health and safety law could potentially breach this Act, although the severity of the breach would be considered, e.g. serious neglect; reckless disregard for health and safety requirements; repeated breaches which create significant risks; false information and serious risks which have been deliberately created to increase profit.

Common Law of Negligence

The common law of negligence asserts that everyone owes a duty of care which requires one to consider the consequences of their acts and omissions and to ensure that those acts and/or omissions do not give rise to a foreseeable risk of injury to any other person.

In simple terms, it requires everyone to owe a duty not to injure other people by our negligent acts and omissions, and this is an individual duty which each of us owes all of the time to our 'neighbours', or those we are providing a service to. Obviously the relevance of this to equipment provision is quite broad, but does, however, fit into almost every part of service delivery and commissioning.

A duty of care can be owed by both individual practitioners and also by organisations as a whole. In addition to their own duty of care, organisations will also be vicariously liable for the negligent acts of employees.

> **POTENTIAL LEGAL BREACHES**
> An example of a breach might be a serious untoward incident that occurs, because the service provider failed to maintain equipment in accordance with manufacturer's instructions.

Consumer Protection Act 1987 (Part 1)

Part 1 of the Consumer Protection Act 1987 transposes the Product Liability Directive (85/374/EEC and 1999/34/EC) into UK law. The legislation imposes strict liability on producers for harm caused by defective products.

The legislation applies to all consumer products and products used at a place of work.

The direct application to equipment providers might be where it manufactures products, e.g. banisters.

> **POTENTIAL LEGAL BREACHES**
>
> There would be a case for breach of the Act where a product manufactured by an equipment provider had a defect with the potential to cause harm.
>
> There may also be a case against equipment providers if they modified equipment, which subsequently was issued with a defect in it, without first consulting the original manufacturer or following their guidance.

General Product Safety Regulations 2005

According to the Department for Business Enterprise and Regulatory Reform (BERR), in principle, the 2005 regulations apply to all products (new and second-hand) used by consumers, whether intended for them or not.

The regulations recognise that products which meet certain other recognised standards, such as relevant British Standards, carry a presumption of conformity with the general safety requirement, meaning that products that comply with them are deemed to be safe.

> **POTENTIAL LEGAL BREACHES**
>
> An obvious breach would be issuing unsafe products into the community, e.g. issuing equipment with exposure to electrical parts, walking frames that break easily, beds or chairs with exposure to entrapment. Buying products which meet British or International Safety Standards may not necessarily be sufficient protection, especially for items which are reissued to another user.

Manual Handling Operations Regulations 1992

This applies to any aspect of the service where manual handling arises.

In an equipment provider setting this could be within a store, during delivery, installation, or maintenance, or a user or carer using the equipment. For example, often heavy equipment is required upstairs in people's homes, e.g. beds, hoists.

The employer, usually the equipment provider, will be responsible for ensuring all manual handling risks to staff are avoided, where possible, which could otherwise result in injury. Both the commissioner and provider could be held responsible for injury to a service user or carer. There should be appropriate risk assessments and governance arrangements in place, together with processes for monitoring and reviewing these assessments on an ongoing basis.

Ideally these arrangements should be set out within the service specification.

Where equipment is provided to reduce the risks involved in manual handling, e.g. hoists, slings, trolleys, etc., it should go without saying that adequate training, information and instructions on the use of the equipment must be provided. Merely providing such equipment (and any necessary training) will not absolve an employer from further responsibility or from liability: use of the equipment should be monitored and encouraged.

POTENTIAL LEGAL BREACHES

A serious breach of these regulations might occur where, for example, a driver is injured delivering an item such as a bed single-handedly, when it should have been a two-person task. The case would be strengthened if there was no evidence of risk assessments or governance arrangements in place for monitoring and assessing risks.

To avoid a breach there would need to be evidence to demonstrate:

- attempts have been made to avoid the manual handling operation, so far as is reasonably practicable
- where manual handling cannot be avoided, a suitable and sufficient risk assessment is carried out, factoring in the task,

---

working environment, the physical capabilities of the individuals involved, and other relevant factors
- appropriate steps have been taken to reduce the risk to health to the lowest level reasonably practicable.

Medical Devices Regulations 2002 (Amended 2003)

These regulations require certain duties to be followed by manufacturers of equipment in particular, e.g. performance and safety standards, CE Marking. There could be application to equipment provision where a provider manufactures equipment, e.g. banisters, and where they modify CE-marked equipment.

POTENTIAL LEGAL BREACHES

Example breaches could be:

- manufacturing a sub-standard product
- adapting or modifying certain pieces of equipment
- acquiring equipment inappropriately, e.g. not CE marked.

Sale and Supply of Goods and Services Act 1982 and Sale and Supply of Goods Act 1994

The Sale and Supply of Goods and Services Act 1982 requires a supplier of a service to carry out that service with reasonable care and skill and, unless agreed to the contrary, within a reasonable time and make no more than a reasonable charge.

Both of the Acts above require that any goods supplied must be as described, of satisfactory quality and fit for their purpose. If they are not, the consumer is entitled to a repair, replacement or compensation.

A claim can be pursued through the courts for up to six years providing it can be shown that the problem was due to the work not being carried out properly or the goods or materials used not being of satisfactory quality.

Equipment supplied to a service user could potentially class as a 'supply of goods' and the fitting of a product into a service user's home could be a 'supply of services'.

The Acts could also be applicable where there are top-ups, direct payments or prescriptions issued by equipment providers, or indeed where equipment is sold directly from a provider to the service user.

POTENTIAL LEGAL BREACHES

There could be a breach if equipment providers did not carry out fitting services with reasonable care and skill. It goes without saying that all equipment issued should be of good quality and fit for purpose.

Where services use top-ups, personal budgets, vouchers or prescriptions, responsibility may lie with the commissioner to ensure service standards are specified.

MHRA Managing Medical Devices DB2006 (05) November 2006

In relation to the provision of equipment, this is perhaps the most informative and comprehensive piece of guidance produced to date. It covers all aspects of managing medical devices. It also sets out recommended processes and directly refers to pertinent legislation, e.g. health and safety, consumer protection.

In the unfortunate event of an untoward incident, serious or fatal accident, relating to any aspect of a medical device, it is very likely service standards would be investigated in line with the principles set out in this guidance.

A serious breach of this guidance could potentially result in gross negligence or failed duty of care.

This guidance should be in the possession of every commissioning authority, and all providers of equipment services.

POTENTIAL LEGAL BREACHES

This is a comprehensive and explicit piece of guidance which has been made available for the specific purpose of managing medical devices. The guidance covers almost all aspects of medical device management relating to equipment services, and various other assistive technologies.

There are numerous ways in which the regulations surrounding how equipment is 'managed' – acquired, stored, recycled, maintained, issued, etc. – could be breached, if any aspect of the guidance was not followed, particularly by an equipment provider. Commissioners could also be held responsible for not having adequate measures in place to manage devices appropriately, such as failing to have a Medical Device Management Board in place, for example. Appendix 5 contains further information about the subject of managing medical devices.

Lifting Operations and Lifting Equipment Regulations 1998 (LOLER)

Lifting equipment is defined as 'work equipment for lifting or lowering loads and includes attachments for anchoring, fixing or supporting it'.

These regulations have a huge impact upon equipment providers as a significant number of equipment categories fall under the LOLER remit, e.g. hoists, stairlifts.

In many service areas there is great ambiguity around what should and what should not be subject to regular LOLER examination, e.g. beds, bathlifts. One approach to determine whether equipment used at work is an item of lifting equipment or not, would be the 'primary purpose' test; for instance, hoists and lifts are clearly lifting equipment, whereas an adjustable-height bed is probably primarily a bed and only secondarily lifting equipment.

Clearly there will be grey areas and, ultimately it would be for the courts to decide what is, and what is not, lifting equipment. However, all this need not cause equipment and adaptation providers undue concern, since the range of duties required under LOLER for lifting equipment, such as a strict duty of maintenance, also apply to all work equipment under the Provision and Use of Work Equipment Regulations 1998.

Section three of the Health and Safety at Work etc. Act 1974 more generally covers equipment subject to LOLER regulations in the service user's home. Section three would apply in place of LOLER, if the lifting equipment were not being used 'at work', because LOLER only applies in this latter circumstance. For example, if a hoist were being operated by an informal family carer, then it would not be equipment used at work and would fall under section three of the 1974 Act but not under LOLER.

The Lifting Operations and Lifting Equipment Regulations 1998 impose further obligations relating to the examination and inspection, strength and stability, positioning and installation of equipment. There is also very much an overlap with PUWER regulations set out below.

HSE produced guidance on LOLER (2012) entitled, *How the Lifting Operations and Lifting Equipment Regulations apply to health and social care.* This guidance should be consulted for clarity regarding specific aspects of LOLER.

It is recommended to regularly check HSE's website for pertinent and up-to-date guidance as this is often updated: www.hse.gov.uk.

POTENTIAL LEGAL BREACHES
A clear breach of these regulations would be failing to carry out recommended LOLER inspections. It is also important to note that the regulations do not only cover the once or twice a year inspection, but also require such things as ensuring:

• the equipment is of adequate strength and stability for the purpose it is to be used for

---

- the equipment is positioned and installed appropriately
- equipment is marked appropriately with safe working loads, etc.
- equipment defects are reported appropriately.

In the event of an incident, failure to meet the above requirements could also indicate a breach of the regulations.

Provision and Use of Work Equipment Regulations 1998 (PUWER)

PUWER requires all equipment used at work, including by paid carers and clinical staff, etc., to be:

- suitable for the intended use and for conditions in which it is used
- safe, maintained, and inspected to ensure it continues to be safe
- used only by the people who have received adequate information, instruction and training
- accompanied with suitable safety measures, e.g. protective devices, markings, warnings.

It is most likely that the commissioners would have to request compliance with these regulations, and that the provider would be responsible for meeting these.

'The Provision and Use of Work Equipment Regulations 1998 make it the employer's responsibility to ensure that work equipment is so constructed or adapted as to be suitable for the purpose for which it is used or provided. The regulations also impose a strict liability duty to maintain equipment in an efficient state, efficient working order and in good repair.' (www.careandhealthlaw.com – Accessed January 2009)

POTENTIAL LEGAL BREACHES

These regulations make it the employer's responsibility to ensure work equipment is constructed or adapted in order to be suitable for the purpose for which it is used or provided.

Possible breaches might be:

- inappropriate assessments and equipment selection by clinical staff
- equipment not maintained properly with planned preventative maintenance programmes in place
- safety information and warnings not issued with equipment.

Control of Substances Hazardous to Health Regulations 2002 (COSHH)

In addition to the usual requirements within the workplace under this regulation, e.g. the management of chemicals or detergents, equipment providers should strictly adhere to this regulation in relation to the control of biological agents such as bacteria and other dangerous micro-organisms.

This regulation especially relates to infected or contaminated equipment. There should be clear policies and procedures developed to ensure potentially infectious diseases are kept under control, e.g. protective clothing, decontamination/infection control guidance.

POTENTIAL LEGAL BREACHES

A most likely breach would be the failure to comply with COSHH requirements – especially in the event of an untoward incident.

Failing in any of the following areas could result in a breach:

- assessing risks
- deciding on precautions needed
- measures to prevent and control risks
- ensuring control measures are used and maintained
- monitoring exposure and health surveillance
- informing, instructing and training employees about risks and precautions.

It has been argued by some lawyers that COSHH regulations could apply to MRSA and Clostridium Difficile (C Diff) issues – although this may be difficult to prove at present. However, failing to control substances likely to cause infection or contamination would be treading on dangerous ground.

The Reporting of Injuries, Diseases and Dangerous Occurrences Regulations 1995 (RIDDOR)

RIDDOR places a legal duty on employers and people in control of premises to: report work-related deaths, major injuries or over three-day injuries, work-related diseases, and dangerous occurrences (near-miss accidents).

Equipment-related injuries should be reported to the appropriate health and safety coordinator, or medical devices board. Equipment commissioners should ensure appropriate health and safety, risk management and governance arrangements are in place.

POTENTIAL LEGAL BREACHES

An obvious breach of these regulations would be not to have any reporting mechanisms in place for allowing injuries to be reported.

There would also be a serious breach of the regulations if injuries and dangerous occurrences, etc. failed to be reported deliberately, or not.

Appendix 2

Guide for contract management indicators

Note. This section is for guidance only and does not form part of the Code of Practice.

The following information sets out suggested contract management indicators and data which could be used for managing disability equipment, wheelchair and seating services. The indicator or information to assist with contract management is highlighted below in the bold headings, supported by a brief description of what is actually being measured.

Note. The information below does not replace any national or locally agreed indicators.

1. **Reasons for failing to deliver equipment within agreed timescale**

   This information enables commissioners to manage service provision effectively by allowing them to focus on possible areas of weakness – which may be internal or external to the service provider. This information is crucial for effective contract management.

   This information can also include times from referral to assessment, through to the date the decision to supply the equipment was made; or the prescription date for the equipment through to the delivery of equipment.

2. **Waiting lists**

   This shows the number of service users waiting for equipment. It also shows the length of time service users are waiting – particularly those who have fallen outside the performance indicator criteria. A reduction in the waiting lists shows progress in performance.

3. **Stock value, turnaround, write-offs, collection rates and recycling levels**
    These levels will have to be ascertained and agreed locally. Collection rates and recycling levels (where applicable) are most important as these indicate the efficiency of the provider.

4. **Number of assets requiring and being maintained, e.g. PAT and LOLER**
    This helps to assess the performance of the provider; more importantly, it highlights the level of risk to the service user and the organisation.

    Note. Services should look to develop local targets for urgent repairs, e.g. 100% within 24hrs.

5. **Performance measures regarding: supplier performance (lead times etc.); savings achieved; cost-saving strategies through improved recall systems, recycling and improved maintenance scheduling**
    This is in keeping with the overall agenda to provide an economical and efficient service, and one that delivers best value. It informs commissioners how efficient the provider is.

6. **Quality improvement targets including, for example, the number of complaints/compliments; results from service user satisfaction surveys; staff turnover rates; infection control (random spot checks); quality control processes in place, e.g. policies and procedures**
    These measures are important as they determine the quality of the service being provided to the service user. Also, good results for these indicators help to sustain high levels of staff morale, with subsequent low staff turnover, etc.

All of these measures look at the quality outputs of the service from a governance, service user/staff satisfaction and overall provider performance perspective.

Appendix 3

Semta Occupational Standards specifically for equipment technicians

Note. This section is for guidance only and does not form part of the Code of Practice.

Semta Occupational Standard Level 2 (or equivalent)
An individual who has completed Level 2 is assumed to be competent to perform the following tasks:

- Dismantle, remove and replace or repair faulty components, in line with company procedures, on a variety of different types of assistive technology systems and equipment, such as manual and powered wheelchairs, buggies and scooters, postural support systems, hoists, personal communication aids, walking aids, adjustable beds, pressure relief and distribution equipment, telecare alarm systems, aids for daily living, environmental control systems, associated battery charging systems for assistive technology systems and equipment;
- Cover a range of maintenance activities, such as isolating equipment, labelling components, dismantling components to the required level, setting and adjusting components, replacing or repairing components, carrying out functional checks and safety checks before handing over to the end user.

Semta Occupational Standard Level 3 (or equivalent)
An individual who has completed Level 3 is assumed to be competent to carry out the following tasks in addition to those for Level 2:

- Carry out servicing activities on mechanical and electromechanical assistive technology equipment, in accordance with approved procedures;

- Service a range of mechanical/electromechanical assistive technology equipment such as wheelchairs, hoists, stairlifts, seating, walking aids, adjustable beds, pressure redistribution cushions, ramps, and aids to daily living. This may involve dismantling, removing and replacing faulty equipment, at component or unit level, on a variety of different types of assistive-technology equipment;
- Apply a range of dismantling and reassembly methods and techniques, such as mechanical fitting, fixing, fastening, soldering, crimping, harnessing, and securing cables and components;
- Comply with (internal) organisational policy and procedures for the servicing activities undertaken, and report any problems with the activities that cannot be personally resolved, or that are outside permitted authority, to the relevant people;
- Work with minimal supervision, taking personal responsibility for actions and for the quality and accuracy of the work carried out.

Appendix 4

Supporting guidance relating to training on Information Systems and Information Management for individual roles

Note. This section is for guidance only and does not form part of the Code of Practice.

This section sets out, as an example, the level of understanding and training requirements, particularly related to information systems, for the various roles involved in the provision of disability equipment.

Management staff
Service level agreements and contract management reports, stock turnover, trend analysis, stock requisition, audit trails, cost allocation to budgets and virtual budget management, expenditure by referrer, e.g. scheme of delegation, key performance indicator reporting, including mitigation/exclusion reports, recalls including MHRA and HSE warnings and notices, planned maintenance management, satellite store management, waiting list management, mail-shots, batch reporting, user-defined fields, e-procurement, export of data to other software packages, e.g. Excel.

Stores staff, administration, technicians and drivers
Delivery and return requests, recycling, asset management, asset type set-up, service template set-up, asset register, asset service and maintenance (planned maintenance schedule), managing stock levels (set stock alerts), multiple stores capability, process orders, assign stock, pick order, deliver order, and use of hand-held devices, where appropriate.

Prescribers (clinical staff)
Online ordering, online product catalogue viewing, stock information, user instructions, health and safety instructions, detailed product descriptions,

and functions such as: request non-stock item, request a return, track a return, request a repair and track a repair.

Where equipment services are working within a scheme of delegation using a pooled funding arrangement, or alternatively virtual budget management, senior clinical staff might need to be able to create, schedule, view, run and understand expenditure and activity reports.

Appendix 5

Supporting guidance relating to Medical Device Management

Note. This section does not form part of the Code of Practice, but should be considered when developing policy or assessing compliance with medical device management issues.

For full details relating to medical device management see: MHRA (2006). *Managing Medical Devices. Guidance for healthcare and social services organisations.* DB2006 (05), only available on website: www.mhra.gov.uk.

Policies and procedures
In relation to equipment provision, the Medical Device Management Group, or appropriate partnership or commissioning board, will have in place policies that address the following topics:

Note. This list is not exhaustive.

- decontamination procedures
- procurement arrangements
- records, both manual and electronic
- adverse incident reporting, including responsible individuals
- actions required on MHRA's medical device alerts and manufacturers' corrective notices
- a named medical device lead with responsibility for responding to alerts
- training on use, assembly, installation, cleaning and disposal
- technical specifications

- regulatory compliance and related issues, e.g. Provision and Use of Work Equipment Regulations (PUWER).

Reporting incidents

MHRA rely on incidents relating to medical devices being reported by local agencies. When sufficient incidents have been reported, MHRA may send out a public alert. It is most important, therefore, that individual organisations take this responsibility seriously, and that they have systems and processes in place which allow this to happen.

According to MHRA, information from adverse incident reporting suggests that factors having the greatest impact on the safety of devices involve the instructions issued by the manufacturer, their availability and clarity, the design of equipment, the quality of training in the appropriate uses of devices and how well they are maintained and prepared.

The causes of incidents may include:

- inadequate instructions for use from the manufacturer
- poor training
- problems arising from the design or manufacturing process
- inappropriate local modifications or adjustments
- inadequate maintenance
- inadequate or inappropriate repairs or replacement parts
- unsuitable storage or use conditions
- inadequate end-of-life or scrapping information.

Failings relating to any of the above can result in very serious incidents. It is important that when incidents are reported, the reason is provided.

Medical Devices Management Board (or overseeing group)

There should be a Medical Devices Management Board (MDMB), or overseeing group, in place to develop and implement policies across the organisation. These will usually review the various medical device policies at least once a year. It is essential that a member of the MDMB represents the interests of equipment services. It is also essential that any medical device-related policy or procedure is endorsed by the MDMB. There should be adequate information networks in place to enable communication to and from the MDMB. Individuals involved should include: service/store managers; technical staff; purchasing staff; clinical professionals.

Although much of this activity will be covered by internal audit teams, as part of the organisation's governance and risk management arrangements, it is essential that equipment provision is represented on the MDMB.

Acquisition processes

A fundamental part of medical device management is in the acquisition of equipment. It is easy to assume that products are safe and of good quality just because they are sold or loaned from reputable suppliers.

Where one exists, the Medical Devices Management Group, or product selection group, should have local policies for the acquisition of medical devices to address safety, quality, and performance as well as all aspects of the acquisition cycle. Policies should include and take account of the needs and preferences of all interested parties, e.g. those involved in use, commissioning, purchasing, decontamination, maintenance and decommissioning. Policies will also factor in local and national acquisition policies, whole-life costs, the method of acquisition, e.g. purchasing and/or leasing.

Where equipment is either on loan, trial or for assessment purposes, it must be clear whose responsibility it will be should any problems arise.

In-house manufacture

Provider services that manufacture medical devices, e.g. banisters or ramps, but do not place them on the market, should only do so in accordance with the Medical Devices Regulations – MHRA DB2006 (05).

Modifying and changing use

Modifying existing devices or using them for purposes not intended by the manufacturer (off-label use) has safety implications, especially in the event of an adverse incident. It may also count as manufacture of a new device under the Medical Devices Regulations, according to MHRA. Those undertaking modifications or changing the use of equipment should only do so in accordance with Medical Devices Regulations – MHRA DB2006 (05). Modifications in use outside of the manufacturer's intended use will only be considered as part of a fully documented risk management process within the provider service risk management policy and procedures.

There are some organisations with the necessary specialist skills and experience for modifying and changing the use of equipment, so that the needs of service users with specific requirements can be met. For example, Remap is a charity, working through a nationwide network of dedicated volunteers to provide this type of service. Remap's unique pieces of special equipment are tailor-made and given free to the people who need them. Remap already has eighty-five panels across England, Wales and Northern Ireland, and helps over 3,000 people with disabilities each year. For further information visit: www.remap.org.uk.

Where modifications are made to equipment or changing its use, the following factors should be considered:

Fitness for intended purpose/application
- Whether the device is compatible with other devices, and any medicinal products that it is likely to be used with.
- Whether the manufacturer intends the device to be used by those who will be using it.
- Whether the device is appropriate for the intended environment.

Safety and performance
- Does the equipment have a suitable CE mark, ISO Standard?
- Is there evidence of historic problems with the equipment?
- Do MHRA safety publications, manufacturer's advisory notices or other relevant publications identify issues related to the device?

Maintenance support services
- Can the equipment service provider (in-house or contractor) maintain the equipment?
- Is alternative equipment available to cover periods when equipment is being repaired or serviced?
- Are response times appropriate and guaranteed?

- What are the proposed intervals between service, and the frequency and complexity of checks?

Training
The need for training depends upon the equipment and can involve users, carers or staff:
- Will it be required for all anticipated users, carers or staff?
- Will it be required for maintenance and repair staff, to enable them to carry out these aspects?

Technical support
- Does the manufacturer give free access to technical advice?
- Is there a 24-hour helpline?
- Is there a troubleshooting list supplied with equipment?

Support services
- Is the installation to be carried out by manufacturer/supplier?
- What building and utility services are required?
- Is special decontamination or calibration needed?
- What other associated equipment is needed?

Second-hand equipment
Usage and service history should always be available for prospective purchasers before sale and then supplied with the equipment at the point of sale. As a minimum there should be a:

- record of any reconditioning work carried out, including a record of replacement parts
- copy of all maintenance and servicing that has been carried out, including the name of maintenance/servicing organisation, and a record of usage and decontamination status.

Electrical safety testing (portable appliance testing)
The provider's medical device management policy should cover the provision of maintenance and repair of all medical devices, including reconditioning and refurbishment. This should include, for example:

- how each category of equipment should be maintained and repaired, and by whom
- the timescale for planned preventative maintenance, e.g. full service every twelve months and a visual inspection every six months
- the timescale for repairs to be completed, e.g. urgent repairs to be dealt with within twelve hours
- the frequency and type of planned preventive maintenance should be specified, taking account of the manufacturer's instructions, the expected usage and the environment in which it is to be used.

Training for professional and end users
Medical device policy should clearly set out the training requirements for professional users, e.g. therapist, and the user, e.g. service user or carer.

Professional users
Professional users need to understand how the manufacturer intends the device/equipment to be used, and how it works normally, to be able to use it effectively and safely.

Where relevant, professional users should:

- be aware of differences between models, and compatibility with other products
- be able to fit accessories
- be able to use any controls appropriately
- understand any displays, indicators, alarms, etc.
- be aware of cleaning and decontamination requirements
- demonstrate how to use the product
- understand the importance of reporting device-related adverse incidents to the MHRA.

End users
End users, i.e. service users or carers, need to understand the intended use and normal functioning of the device in order to use it effectively and safely.

Where relevant, training for end users should cover:

- limitations on use
- how to fit accessories
- how to use any controls appropriately
- explanation of displays, indicators, alarms, etc. and how to respond to them
- explanation of requirements for maintenance and decontamination; how to recognise when the device is not working properly and what to do about it, e.g. troubleshoot
- explanation of the importance of reporting device-related adverse incidents to the MHRA.

Information, record management and manufacturers' instructions
It is crucial that all of the information relating to medical device management is coordinated, centrally controlled, and kept in a safe and accessible location. Good record keeping is essential for the safe management of medical devices. Often a significant amount of information relating specifically to equipment can be held electronically in the disability equipment service's IT system.

Information held electronically will play a crucial part when conducting planned maintenance schedules, or when carrying out a product recall. It is important to ensure information held against products is valid and up to date. This would be particularly important should an investigation take place following an untoward incident.

Some IT systems for managing equipment are quite advanced and are capable of assisting with most aspects of medical device management. For example, they can hold manufacturers' information, which can be downloaded by professional and end users. They are also capable of sending out medical device alerts to professional users.

It is also important to ensure approved protocols are followed when deleting information. It may be necessary to have archive arrangements in place. This should be reflected in local policy.

As can be seen, careful consideration should be given to information management and record keeping, and should be clearly set out within the medical device management policy for the provision of equipment.

Audit and review

Random internal quality audits and reviews should be carried out on all elements of maintenance and repair to ensure that the correct procedures are in place and that they are being adhered to.

Decontamination and disposal processes

Disposal of equipment is an area which does not generally receive much attention, but given the potential for associated cross-contamination risks, a safe disposal process is essential. Some issues which need to be factored in when considering this process include:

- The expected life cycle of a piece of equipment, i.e. should certain pieces of equipment be disposed of after certain periods?
- Development of replacement criteria, e.g. whether the equipment is damaged or worn out beyond economic repair, poor reliability, clinical or technical obsolescence, changes in local policies for device use, absence of manufacturer/supplier support, non-availability of correct replacement parts, non-availability of specialist repair knowledge, users' opinions, possible benefits of new model (features, usability, more clinically effective, lower running costs), or the life cycle of the medical device.
- Manufacturers should provide the best methods of waste disposal. They should be able to provide details of the current techniques and processes applicable to their products.
- Where applicable, equipment should be decontaminated before disposal, and supplied with a certificate of decontamination.
- When transporting equipment, arrangements will need to be in place to ensure that it is appropriately packaged and secured. The Carriage of Dangerous Goods by Road Regulations 1996 legislation applies to the safe transport of goods by road. It is of equal importance to ensure that consideration is given to disposal arrangements for third-party contractors. It should also not be expected for professional users or end users to dispose of contaminated equipment in their cars, or put contaminated and soiled equipment in household bins.
- Decommissioning aims to make equipment safe and unusable, while minimising damage to the environment and to individuals. Any equipment deemed unfit for reuse should be decommissioned.

Decommissioning should include decontamination, making safe, and making unusable. This is to ensure that an inappropriate person does not use the equipment and expose themselves to potential hazards.

The above points highlight the necessity for decontamination and disposal issues to be clearly documented in an equipment medical device management policy.

Appendix 6

Supporting guidance relating to the choice of decontamination method appropriate to the degree of infection risk associated with the intended use of the equipment

This information was taken from MHRA *Managing Medical Devices* document (MHRA DB2006 (05) November 2006). Accessible on MHRA website only.

Classification of infection risk associated with the decontamination of medical devices

Risk	Application of Item	Recommendation
High	In close contact with broken skin or broken mucous membrane. Introduced into sterile body areas.	Cleaning followed by sterilization.
Medium	In contact with mucous membranes. Contaminated with particularly virulent or readily transmissible organisms. Before use on immunocompromised patients.	Cleaning followed by sterilization or disinfection. NB: Where sterilization will damage equipment, cleaning followed by high-level disinfection may be used as an alternative.
Low	In contact with healthy skin. Not in contact with patient.	Cleaning.

Other factors to consider when choosing a method of decontamination include the:

- nature of the contamination
- time required for processing
- heat, pressure, moisture and chemical tolerance of the item
- availability of the processing equipment
- quality and risks associated with the decontamination method.

Appendix 7

Glossary

assessment: evaluation of an individual's need by a person who is professionally qualified and approved to do so.

assistive technology: product, device or service designed to enable independence for disabled or older people.

carer: any person, paid or unpaid, who undertakes a caring role for a service user.

clinical services interface: aspects of clinical responsibilities that interface with disability equipment services.

commissioner: individual within local authority, NHS, or other public service, appointed to be responsible for the strategic level process of planning, specifying, securing and monitoring services to meet people's needs.

complex, specialist and children's equipment: items of disability equipment which are not generally classified as standard or routine equipment.

Note. These items will typically be complex by design and may be bespoke or specially adapted or tailored to meet the particular needs of the individual for whom they are prescribed.

continuing healthcare equipment: equipment supplied to a person who has been accepted as having continuing healthcare needs.

cross-border protocol: protocol used to provide guidance relating to the provision of disability equipment across geographic boundaries or partnership borders.

direct payments: money given to service users to enable them to purchase equipment (or services) themselves.

disabled facilities grants: grants provided by local authorities to help meet the cost of adapting a property for the needs of a disabled person.

eligibility criteria: level of assessment of need to which an organisation will seek to provide services.

minor adaptations: minor alterations made to a service user's property.

> *Note.* Minor adaptations are for the purpose of increasing or maintaining functional independence to enable the service user to remain in their own home, to ensure safety and/or to assist carers by minimising the physical demands placed on them.

partnership board: the structure for the management and planning of the provision of a disability equipment service across a number of partner organisations in one geographical area.

person-centred care: sees patients as equal partners in planning, developing and assessing care to make sure it is most appropriate for their needs. It involves putting patients and their families at the heart of all decisions.

personal budget: a sum of money allocated to people as a result of an assessment of their needs. The amount of money people are awarded is based on the 'eligible needs' they have at that time. Eligible needs are those which the local council's policy says it has a duty to support people with.

personal health budget: an amount of money to support a person's health and wellbeing needs, planned and agreed between the person and their local NHS team.

prescriber: person permitted by one of the purchasing authorities to assess a service user's need for an adaptation or equipment, and to requisition the item from the equipment service.

provider: organisation or individual responsible for supplying the specified equipment services on behalf of the purchasing or commissioning authorities.

recycling: retrieval, cleaning and decontamination, maintenance, repair and refurbishment, so that equipment is fit for reissue.

requisition: formal order request for disability equipment.

self-assessment: service user assessing their own needs and, where appropriate, selecting their own items of disability equipment.

service user: person who requires and uses disability equipment or adaptations supplied by the service following a needs assessment.

social model of disability: model focusing on structures and their barriers which disabled individuals experience (for example, inaccessible transport, housing and education provision) and provides tools for dismantling and preventing these.

Note. This contrasts with the medical model, which looks at medical impairments as the main reason for difficulties experienced by disabled people.

trusted assessor: staff such as assistants and support workers who have undergone specific training to assess people requiring disability equipment, usually in relation to 'straightforward' and low-risk needs.